The Best Boring Book Ever of

Select Healthcare Classification Systems and Databases

by

Katherine S. Rowell
and Ann Cutrell

The Best Boring Book Ever of
Select Healthcare Classification Systems and Databases

ISBN 978-0-615-90976-9

Designed by:

Breviloquent
Lexington, Massachusetts | Charlottesville, Virginia
www.breviloquent.com

More information:

www.healthdataviz.com

Acknowledgments

Without the following people's expertise, sage guidance, and good old fashioned hard work, this book would never have seen the light of day.

There were two women named Ann[e] (one with an "e" and one without)—my comrades in arms throughout this project—both of whom I am grateful and proud to call my friends.

The first is my former student and co-author, Ann Cutrell, who was tireless in finding and compiling the material needed for this book. What started out as "only" a research role quickly turned into shared authorship. Without her unflagging dedication, this book would still just be a good idea rolling around in my head.

The second Anne is "GrammarLady" (or GL, as we call her). I met GL when I was a student in her adult-education course, "Right Grammar, Right Now." After two sessions, I dropped out and hired her: I know real brains and talent when I see them. There was no way I was ever going to be able to edit my own work with the speed, skill, and humor that she could. Thank you, GL—you did a truly amazing job, and kept me from those horribly embarrassing dangling participles.

I also want to thank the guys at Breviloquent, Jim Leightheiser and Peter Massarelli, for the beautiful design and layout of the book. When I first saw it I literally grinned from ear to ear and jumped up and down. The content may be boring; the design is anything but.

And a final thanks to Stephen Few for encouraging me to pursue this work and to march to my own drummer, and to my husband, Bret, who wondered what took me so long.

ii

Contents

Preface

As you have probably already guessed by the title, this book is not a page-turner; there are no life-changing secrets buried here. Rather, it is meant to serve as a resource for both seasoned professionals in and newcomers to the healthcare industry, a resource that provides concise but thorough descriptions of select clinical classification systems and select healthcare databases.

We have followed a very simple format. Each entry on a named system or database presents a general description of its current state, followed by a timeline of key points in its evolution. Finally, a summary section describes present structure and terminology. This arrangement will, we hope, help the reader understand the antecedents and evolution of these systems and databases, and thereby help guide the choice of exactly the right such resources for a particular project. Which systems and databases align best with the questions you hope to answer, the information you hope to impart? The information presented here should make those decisions and selections faster, easier, smoother, and more confident.

I thought that I knew a lot about finding and using healthcare information and data when we started work on this book, and I was right. As is so often the case, I also came to learn a whole lot more about it than I'd ever imagined I would. I hope you will as well.

Select
Classification Systems

Introduction: Select Classification Systems

Well-defined and widely accepted classification systems for types of illnesses, conditions, treatments, and outcomes of care, along with other dimensions of care such as payment for services and geographic locations of healthcare services and patients demographics, are essential to being able to capture, report, examine, and compare healthcare information throughout the continuum of care.

Deciding on a set of terms (terminology) that accurately represent a system of concepts; creating a vocabulary with definitions of those terms; and arranging and organizing related entities into a classification system would appear to be a fairly straightforward (if long and detailed) task. Well, as the old joke goes, if you want 12 different opinions, put six people in a room and go around twice. (If they're experts in the field, the total will be closer to 24.) Reaching consensus on how to classify healthcare information is tough. Evidence changes; treatments and procedures and patients metamorphose; stakeholders define terms differently based on ever-shifting goals and objectives. All these transformations mean that the way information is defined and classified is continually evolving.

In this section of the book, we describe and document—taking this widespread mutability into account as fully as we can—select healthcare classification systems that are by and large well established, and widely accepted and used. We also cover a few systems that are still finding their way, but are nevertheless relevant, and will we trust be useful to our readers.

Acute Physiology and Chronic Health Evaluation (APACHE®)

Acute Physiology and Chronic Health Evaluation (APACHE®) is a severity-adjusted methodology that predicts outcomes through a scoring system for critically ill adult patients. The system is recognized worldwide as the premier decision-support methodology for adult critical care populations. APACHE® Foundations is a free, web-based offering from Cerner Corporation.

System Evolution

1978   A team led by Dr. William A. Knaus and advised by biostatistician Jerome Cornfield began to develop a clinically based conceptual mathematic model that combined existing clinical knowledge with newer computer-based statistical search techniques to monitor the process and evaluate the outcomes of care. Three years later, the first article to introduce "APACHE," an acronym chosen to stand for the system's major components—acute physiology, age, and chronic health evaluation—was released.

1985   APACHE was remarkably accurate in its ability to risk-stratify patients and to accurately predict mortality rates across institutions and even international boundaries, leading to a second version, APACHE II, which simplified the system. It reduced the number of physiologic measurements required from 33 to 12, and more precisely represented the complex interactions of disease and severity and their effect on a patient's prognosis.

1988   A company based on APACHE, APACHE Medical Systems, Inc. (AMSI), was founded. AMSI was designed to support users of APACHE while providing a more formal structure for researchers.

4

1991   A method to compute a refined score, known as APACHE III scoring, was validated using APACHE data about 17,440 adult medical/surgical intensive care unit (ICU) admissions at 40 U.S. hospitals. This scoring improved the precision of the system by looking at 27 variables (among them diagnosis, age, vital signs, and laboratory values) for each patient.

2001   Integration of electronic data-collection efforts within ICUs was still a slow and fragmented process, contributing to the sale of AMSI to Cerner Corporation, a healthcare information company.

2004   New developments in protocols and practices within ICUs after the launch of APACHE III prompted a full review, updating of all APACHE III equations, resulting in the creation of APACHE IV. Version IV provides risk prediction for outcomes such as mortality and ICU length of stay.

Structure & Terminology

APACHE methodology relies upon a standard set of measures captured on the patient's first day in the ICU to generate the following scores and predictions:

» APS (Acute Physiology Score)

» APACHE III score

» APACHE IV hospital mortality risk prediction

» APACHE IV expected ICU Length of Stay (LOS) prediction

» APACHE II score (for patients with a diagnosis of sepsis)

» Risk-Adjusted Patient List Report

» Aggregated Risk Adjustment Outcomes Report

The system may be used as an on-line calculator to quickly obtain scores and predictions for individual patients or

The APACHE system is recognized worldwide as the premier **decision-support methodology** for adult critical care populations.

subsets of patients or as a severity-adjusted outcomes measurement system for an individual ICU (or group of ICUs) to assess quality of care and identify opportunities for improvement.

Variable	Scoring Range		
Physiology	0-252	.... **Acute Physiology Score (APS)**	
Chronic Health	0-23	⊕ Total ... **Physiologic Reserve**	⊕ Total = **APACHE III Score**
Age	0-24	*(Range = 0-47)*	*(Range = 0-299)*

American Society of Anesthesiologists (ASA) Physical Status Classification System

The American Society of Anesthesiologists (ASA) classification system has been used for decades by anesthetists worldwide as an assessment of the pre-operative physical status of patients prior to selecting an anesthetic or to performing surgery. This score has also been used in policy-making, performance evaluation, and resource allocation of anesthesia services, and is frequently cited in clinical research. The ASA system is not intended as a means of predicting operative risk.

System Evolution

1940   The ASA classification of physical status was introduced by a committee of three physicians: Meyer Saklad, M.D., Emery Rovenstine, M.D., and Ivan Taylor, M.D., to make tabulation of statistical data in anesthesia easier. More particularly, the classification was created to clarify connections between and among the patient's pre-operative condition; the surgical procedure; and outcomes.

1963   ASA reduced the number of original categories, and adopted the five-category physical status classification system; a sixth category was later added.

> The ASA classification is **often misused** as a measure of operative risk, which is the basis of much criticism.

7

Structure & Terminology

» ASA Physical Status 1 - A normal, healthy patient

» ASA Physical Status 2 - A patient with mild systemic disease

» ASA Physical Status 3 - A patient with severe systemic disease

» ASA Physical Status 4 - A patient with severe systemic disease that is a constant threat to life

» ASA Physical Status 5 - A moribund patient who is not expected to survive without the operation

» ASA Physical Status 6 - A declared brain-dead patient whose organs are being removed for donor purposes

» The letter "E" is added following the status number if the surgery is an emergency (except that there is no "6E").

The ASA classification system is a valuable assessment tool that subjectively categorizes patients into subgroups by pre-operative physical fitness prior to administering anesthesia. It was designed originally as a standardized way for physicians to convey information about the patient's overall health status and allow outcomes to be stratified by a global assessment of their severity of illness. However, in practice, the ASA classification is often misused as a measure of operative risk, which is the basis of much criticism.

Apgar Score (APGAR)

The Apgar Score (APGAR) refers to a scoring system used to describe the condition of the newborn infant immediately after birth and, when properly applied, is a tool for standardized assessment. The five categories observed are the baby's color, heart rate, reflexes, muscle tone, and respiratory effort.

System Evolution

1952   Dr. Virginia Apgar, an anesthesiologist, developed a scoring mechanism to evaluate the effects of obstetric anesthesia on babies after delivery. Her system enabled a quick, efficient, simple, and accurate method of assessing clinical status at 1 minute of age, and of gauging the need for prompt intervention to establish breathing. The score report was first presented at a scientific meeting, and later published in 1953.

1958   A second report, evaluating a larger number of patients, was published, and provided a standardized assessment for infants after delivery.

1989   Dr. Joseph Butterfield created the mnemonic APGAR as a way to recall the five scoring criteria: Appearance (skin color), Pulse (heart rate), Grimace (reflex irritability), Activity (muscle tone), and Respiration.

Structure & Terminology

Each criterion is scored 0, 1, or 2 with a maximum final total score of ten. The score is now reported at 5 minutes as well as 1 minute after birth. Scores 3 and below are generally regarded as critically low, 4 to 6 fairly low, and 7 to 10 generally normal.

Dr. Virginia Apgar, an anesthesiologist, developed a scoring mechanism to evaluate the effects of **obstetric anesthesia** on babies after delivery.

9

Heart rate:

» 0 No heart rate

» 1 <100 beats per minute (indicates that the baby is not very responsive)

» 2 >100 beats per minute (indicates that the baby is vigorous)

Respiration:

» 0 Not breathing

» 1 Weak or irregular cry, whimpering, grunting

» 2 Good, strong cry

Muscle tone:

» 0 Limp

» 1 Some flexing or bending of arms and legs

» 2 Active motion

Reflex response:

» 0 No response to airways being stimulated

» 1 Grimace during stimulation

» 2 Grimace and cough or sneeze during stimulation

Color:

» 0 The baby's entire body is blue or pale

» 1 Good color in body, but with blue hands or feet

» 2 Completely pink or good color

The 1-minute Apgar score measures how well the newborn tolerated the birthing process. The 5-minute Apgar score assesses how well the newborn is adapting to the environment and informs medical interventions.

APGAR Scoresheet

Sign	0	1	2	1 min	5 min	10 min	15 min	20 min
A (skin color)	Blue or Pale	Acrocyanotic	Completely pink					
P (heart rate)	Absent	<100 minute	>100 minute					
G (reflex irritability)	No Response	Grimace	Cry or Active Withdrawal					
A (muscle tone)	Limp	Some Flexion	Active Motion					
R (respiration)	Absent	Weak Cry: Hypoventilation	Good, crying					

GESTATIONAL AGE _____ weeks   TOTAL SCORE

11

Current Procedural Terminology (CPT®)

urrent Procedural Terminology (CPT®) is a uniform medical nomenclature that describes medical, surgical, and diagnostic services. The CPT classification system is maintained and updated annually by the American Medical Association (AMA), which holds copyright on it.

System Evolution

1966   CPT was created and introduced by the AMA to standardize terminology among physicians, simplify medical record-keeping, and capture information for actuarial and statistical analysis.

1970s   CPT was expanded to include laboratory procedures. A method of periodically updating its codes was established.

1980s   The Health Care Financing Administration (HCFA), now the Centers for Medicare and Medicaid Services (CMS), merged CPT with its own Healthcare Common Procedure Coding System (HCPCS), and mandated the use of CPT for all Medicare and Medicaid billing.

1990s   The 1996 Health Insurance Portability and Accountability Act (HIPAA) mandated the creation of a single coding system in the United States. To ensure that CPT would be selected as the national standard, the AMA initiated the CPT 5 Project to address perceived deficiencies in the existing system that it would replace.

2000   The Secretary of Health and Human Services (HHS) selected CPT as the national standard. Individual codes were added and others were enhanced to reflect the expanding scope of medical technology and clinical practice.

Structure & Terminology

» **Category I.** These codes describe a procedure or service consistent with contemporary medical practice and are widely performed using a five-digit number and a descriptor; for example, "71010 – Single View Chest" or "62270 – Spinal puncture, lumbar, diagnostic." Category I has six main sub-sections:

    a. Evaluation and Management

    b. Anesthesia

    c. Surgery

    d. Radiology

    e. Pathology & Laboratory

    f. Medicine

» **Category II.** These codes are alphanumeric (four digits and an alpha character), supplemental tracking codes; for example, "3014F — Screening mammography results documented and reviewed." Category II codes capture quality data on patient care.

» **Category III.** These are temporary codes for the reporting and tracking of new and emerging procedures and technologies. They capture data as part of the Food and Drug Administration (FDA) approval process, and substantiate widespread use of new equipment or clinical procedures before permanent codes have been established for these.

CPT® is the most widely accepted **medical nomenclature used to report medical procedures and services** under public and private health insurance programs. The AMA holds copyright in CPT and use or reprinting of CPT in any product or publication requires a license.

Diagnosis-Related Groups (DRG)

Diagnosis-Related Groups (DRG) is the name of a classification system that provides a clinically coherent set of patient classes connecting a hospital's case mix to the resource consumption and associated costs it incurs. DRG are assigned on a case-by-case basis using computer programs called "groupers." Groupers build on information about diagnoses (based on the International Classification of Diseases, or ICD, system), procedures performed, patient age, patient gender, discharge status, and the presence of complications or comorbidities to choose the appropriate group. The Centers for Medicare and Medicaid Services (CMS, formerly the Health Care Financing Administration, HCFA) is responsible for updates to the DRG system; these are published annually on 1 October in the Federal Register.

System Evolution

1975   The DRG system was developed at Yale University for the purpose of grouping patients with similar conditions and treatments for comparative studies.

1983   DRG evolved from a utilization-review system to a tool for reimbursement when HCFA adopted a new method of payment for Medicare inpatient services, the Prospective Payment System (PPS). A PPS is based on prospectively set rates, and thus

DRG evolved from a utilization-review system to a **tool for reimbursement** when HCFA adopted a new method of payment for Medicare inpatient services, the Prospective Payment System (PPS).

represents a change from a cost-based reimbursement system. Under a PPS, each case is categorized into a DRG, which has a payment weight assigned to it based on the average resources used to treat Medicare patients in that DRG. Of the several DRG systems developed so far, the most commonly used is the CMS-DRG.

2007   The biggest change to DRG since its inception occurred with the implementation of Medicare Severity DRG (MS-DRG). CMS began using the new MS-DRG system to better account for differences in the severity of the illness, injury, and|or condition affecting patients.

Structure & Terminology

Numbering system	000-999
Description	The title of each category is the descriptor of that category
Major Diagnostic Category (MDC)	One of 25 systems connected to major organs or etiologies (disease causes)
Type of Code	Medical or Surgical
Weight Assigned	Determined by average resources required to treat a patient, expressed as the baseline relative weight of 1.
Geometric Mean Length of Stay (GMLOS)	Average length of stay for patients in a particular DRG, adjusted to exclude outliers and transferred patients

Arithmetic Mean Length of Stay (AMLOS)	Actual unadjusted length of stay for patients within that DRG
Calculation of Payment Amount	Every hospital is assigned a base rate depending on its location, cost-of-living data, and the severity of illnesses, conditions, and|or injuries treated there. This rate is multiplied by the MS-DRG relative weight (see above, "Weight assigned") to calculate the hospital's payment.

Typically, inpatient facilities use medical billing software to process claims. These billing systems consider the three components of DRG pricing—DRG grouper, weight, and standard base rate—when calculating standard DRG claims payments. Accurate calculations on standard DRG claims depend on a combination of four elements that allow the system to assign the correct DRG groups and weights: surgical procedure codes, diagnosis, patient's age, and patient's gender.

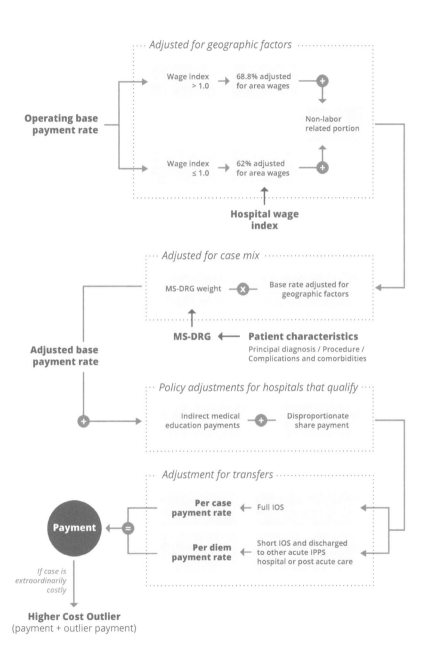

Adjusted for geographic factors

Operating base payment rate

Wage index > 1.0 → 68.8% adjusted for area wages +

Non-labor related portion

Wage index ≤ 1.0 → 62% adjusted for area wages +

Hospital wage index

Adjusted for case mix

MS-DRG weight ✕ Base rate adjusted for geographic factors

MS-DRG ← Patient characteristics
Principal diagnosis / Procedure / Complications and comorbidities

Adjusted base payment rate

Policy adjustments for hospitals that qualify

Indirect medical education payments + Disproportionate share payment

Adjustment for transfers

Per case payment rate ← Full IOS

Payment =

Per diem payment rate ← Short IOS and discharged to other acute IPPS hospital or post acute care

If case is extraordinarily costly

Higher Cost Outlier
(payment + outlier payment)

17

Diagnostic and Statistical Manual of Mental Disorders (DSM)

The Diagnostic and Statistical Manual of Mental Disorders (DSM) is a nomenclature to standardize the diagnostic and coding process for patients with psychiatric disorders. The DSM, often referred to as the "Psychiatrist's Bible," has evolved for use in clinical education and research, for public-health statistics and reimbursement, and by pharmaceutical companies, policy-makers, and courts of law. The American Psychiatric Association (APA) owns the copyright to the DSM; the Division of Research of the Association governs its revision process.

System Evolution

1952   DSM-I: The APA Committee on Nomenclature and Statistics developed a variant of the World Health Organization's International Classification of Diseases-6 (ICD-6, the 1948 version of this nomenclature) because the mental disorder section did not fully meet the needs of the psychiatric profession. This variant was published as the first edition of the DSM. The psychiatric classification organized 106 mental disorders around presumed pathogenic processes.

1968   DSM-II: Even though the APA was involved in the next revision of the mental disorder section of the ICD (version 8), it decided to bring out its own revision, the DSM-II, which listed 182 disorders. These first two versions prescribe diagnostic standards based on psychogenic theory that, in turn, is rooted in psychodynamics.

1980   DSM-III was an innovative solution to address the problem of inter-rater reliability in psychiatric diagnosis; it created a system of explicit, operationalized diagnostic criteria. The psychodynamic emphasis was discarded in favor of a regulatory or legislative model based on objective facts and scientific grounds.

1987   DSM-III-R revised DSM-III, addressing inconsistencies and controversial areas of the latter, and broadening its purview to 292 diagnoses.

1994   The DSM-IV manual provided a tool for clinicians to evaluate patients using a multi-axial system:

> **Axis I:** Clinical disorders, including major mental, learning, and substance-abuse disorders

> **Axis II:** Personality disorders and intellectual disabilities

> **Axis III:** Acute medical conditions and physical disorders

> **Axis IV:** Psychosocial and environmental factors contributing to the disorder

> **Axis V:** Global Assessment of Functioning (GAF), or Children's Global Assessment Scale (for children and teens under 18)

2013   The sweeping revision of DSM-IV, which became DSM-5, has generated extensive controversy, but was nevertheless approved in late 2012 by the American Psychiatric Association.

Hoarding – a psychological condition that can result in homes crammed floor to ceiling with papers, junk mail, books, clothing and other "valuables"— has been associated with **obsessive-compulsive behavior**; although clinical experts have long held that the two disorders aren't necessarily connected.

In the revised, fifth edition of the American Psychiatric Association's Diagnostic and Statistical Manual of Mental Disorders (DSM-5), "hoarding disorder" becomes a separate diagnosis, characterized by a "persistent difficulty discarding or parting with possessions, regardless of their actual value."

These substantial changes, which included a new numbering system, included the folding of Asperger's Syndrome into the broader category of autism spectrum disorder and the inclusion of depression in the bereaved. Other changes include the addition of hoarding and excoriation disorder (compulsive behavior involving constant picking at one's skin).

Structure & Terminology

DSM-5 will abandon the multiaxial system of DSM-IV version and reorder the manual's chapters. The non-axial documentation of diagnosis will combine the former Axes I, II, and III with separate notations for psychosocial and contextual factors (formerly Axis IV) and disability (formerly Axis V). DSM-5's 20 chapters will be restructured based on a new view of disorders' relatedness. These changes will align DSM-5 with the World Health Organization's (WHO) International Classification of Diseases, eleventh edition (ICD-11), and are expected to facilitate improved communication and common use of diagnoses across disorders within chapters.

Geomedicine | Geocoding

Geomedicine is the branch of medicine concerned with the influence of environmental, climactic, and topographic conditions on health and disease prevalence in different parts of the world. Aided by a Geographical Information System (GIS), a patient's exposure to these influences as apparent from her|his place history can be an additional source of information for the clinician during diagnosis and risk-assessment, since geomedicine links the health of a population and the health of an individual through geography.

System Evolution

Pre-1990   The Greek physician Hippocrates (about 400 B.C.) is considered by most scientists to be the founder of medical geology, as he recognized that environmental factors affected the distribution of disease. Much later appeared one of the oldest known examples of disease mapping: a world map of diseases drawn by German physician L.L. Finke in 1792. Other examples of this type of charting include a map by Valentine Seaman of cases of yellow fever in the harbor of New York, published in The Medical Repository in 1798; John Snow's mapping of cholera cases in London (Soho) in 1850; and the French chemist Chatin's observation that the prevalence of goiter varied with the iodine content of the soil of different localities in 1851.

1990-1999   Formal recognition of the sub-discipline appears to reside with H. Ziess, who first introduced the term "geomedicine" in 1931. In 1995, John Wennberg, M.D., inspired and recruited a multi-disciplinary faculty to join him at Dartmouth to explore the questions raised by the variations in medical practice, healthcare spending, and patient outcomes

Geocoding is a primary resource for **data mining** in healthcare, and is quickly becoming the standard for linking data at the local, state, national, and global level.

21

observed in comparisons of individual physicians, populations cared for by hospitals or medical groups, and populations living in different regions of the United States. Known as the Dartmouth Atlas of Health Care Project, this ongoing study has promoted enhanced patient control over care, and fostered improved understanding of the causes and consequences of variation in the way health care is delivered around the United States, thereby supporting accountability for costs and outcomes.

2000s   William Davenhall is noted for concluding that health and geography are inextricably linked, as expressed by his equation "Health = Genetics + Lifestyle + Environment." He has said that geomedicine offers a new type of medical intelligence that takes advantage of national spatial data infrastructures to benefit personal human health and to improve the quality of the care medical professionals deliver. Davenhall advocates place history (a record of every place a person has lived) as a part of the electronic health record (EHR). Ethan Berke, M.D., uses spatial epidemiology and medical geography to understand public health issues such as aging, activity, and obesity, and how they are connected to the built environment as part of his teaching at The Dartmouth Institute (TDI).

Structure & Terminology

Geocoding is the process of converting locations or addresses into geographic coordinates, often latitude and longitude, which can be used to define areas or locations on maps. At a more regional level, location can be found with a postal code, such as a ZIP Code™ in the United States. Computer-based look-up tables that link such postal codes with geocoded coordinates are invaluable when locations become places; that is, when they are charged with meaning. Mapping geographic patterns of cancer incidence and mortality rates in the U.S., pinpointing available health resources, or examining regional differences in the prevalence of asthma can convey far more (and far more valuable) information than can any one element of this type of information alone.

However it is used, geocoding is a primary resource for data mining in healthcare, and is quickly becoming the standard for linking data at the local, state, national, and global level.

Healthcare Common Procedure Coding System (HCPCS)

The Healthcare Common Procedure Coding System (HCPCS, pronounced "hick picks") is a standardized code system used by Medicare and other third-party payers to ensure the consistent processing of claims for medical, surgical, and diagnostic services. Periodic revisions and updates are published on the Centers for Medicare and Medicaid (CMS) website.

System Evolution

1980s — HCPCS was developed by the Health Care Financing Administration (HCFA) governmental agency, now known as the CMS, to provide voluntary standardized coding for items and services provided in the delivery of health care. Initially, there were three levels:

> » Level I or Current Procedural Terminology (CPT-4)
>
> » Level II or HCPCS | National Codes
>
> » Level III or Local Codes

1996 — The implementation of the Health Insurance Portability and Accountability Act (HIPPA) made the use of HCPCS for transactions involving healthcare information mandatory.

Each year, in the United States, healthcare insurers process over **5 billion claims** for payment. For Medicare and other health insurance programs to ensure that these claims are processed in an orderly and consistent manner, standardized coding systems are essential.

HIPPA also required CMS to adopt standards for coding systems, so Level III ("Local") Codes established by insurers and agencies to fulfill local needs were deemed unnecessary, and regulations specified that they be eliminated. Once this deletion occurred, the official name of the classification system was changed to HCPCS Level II Code Set.

2000s   The Secretary of Health & Human Services (HHS) delegated authority under the HIPAA legislation to CMS to maintain and distribute HCPCS Level II Codes. The next year, CMS revised the process it used to update the code sets. This revision was to expedite the decision process for coverage, to allow new technologies to get to patients more quickly.

Structure & Terminology

Level I codes are five-digit numbers using the American Medical Association (AMA)'s Current Procedural Terminology (CPT).

Level II HCPCS codes, which are established by CMS's Alpha-Numeric Editorial Panel, primarily represent items and supplies and non-physician services not covered by the American Medical Association's Current Procedural Terminology-4 (CPT-4) codes, such as ambulance services and durable medical equipment, prosthetics, orthotics, and supplies (DMEPOS) when used outside a physician's office. Medicare, Medicaid, and private health insurers use HCPCS procedure and modifier codes for claims processing. Level II alphanumeric procedure and modifier codes include the A to V range (the HCPCS system does not include every letter in this range).

>> **A Codes:** Transportation Services, including Ambulance and Medical and Surgical Supplies

>> **B Codes:** Enteral and Parenteral Therapy

>> **C Codes:** Outpatient Prospective Payment System (PPS)

>> **D Codes:**   Dental Procedures

>> **E Codes:** Durable Medical Equipment (DME)

>> **G Codes:** Procedures|Professional Services, usually when no CPT exists

» **H Codes:** Alcohol and Drug Abuse Treatment Services

» **J Codes:** Drugs Administered Other than by Oral Method

» **K Codes:** Temporary Codes for Use by DME Medicare Administrative Contractors (MAC's)

» **L Codes:** Orthotic and Prosthetic Procedures and Devices

» **M Codes:** Medical Services that do not qualify for CPT codes

» **P Codes:** Pathology and Laboratory

» **Q Codes:** Temporary

» **R Codes:** Diagnostic Radiology Services

» **S Codes**: Temporary National Codes, Non-Medicare (for example: Home Infusion)

» **T Codes:** Used by state Medicaid and some private insurers

» **V Codes:** Vision and Hearing Services

International Classification of Diseases (ICD)

The International Statistical Classification of Diseases and Related Health Problems (ICD) is the most widely used nosology (systematic classification of diseases); it assigns alphanumeric designations to every diagnosis, description of symptoms, and cause of death attributed to human beings. The use of disease codes from the ICD has expanded from classifying morbidity and mortality information for statistical purposes to diverse sets of applications in research, healthcare policy, and healthcare finance. The ICD is updated and maintained by the World Health Organization.

System Evolution

1893	The first international List of Causes of Death evolved from the Bertillon Classification of Causes of Death, founded by the French physician Jacques Bertillon and listing 179 causes. Subsequently known as the International Classification of Causes of Death (ICD), it was to be revised every 10 years.
1900-1948	Four revisions, from the first ICD to ICD-5, took place over this time period. With each revision, the numbers of codes increased, as did the appeal of using them for other purposes.
1955-1975	Three successive decennial revision conferences recognized the increasing use of ICD for the indexing of hospital medical records for ICD-6 through ICD-8.
1977-1985	ICD-9 was published; work on ICD-10 began.
1996	ICD-10 implementation outside the United States started. The U.S. is bound by international treaty to report mortality data to World Health Organization (WHO) using ICD-10 codes; it began compliance in 1999.

2003   The Health Insurance Portability and Accountability Act (HIPAA) named ICD-9 as the code set for reporting diagnoses and hospital inpatient procedures in electronic administrative transactions. To make the ICD more useful for American hospitals, the National Center for Health Statistics (NCHS) created an extension of it so that the system could be used for morbidity as well as mortality. The classification's name was changed to the International Classification of Diseases, Ninth Revision, Clinical Modification (ICD-9-CM).

2013   The original implementation date for ICD-10-CM in the United States; this implementation was however postponed until 2014. The NCHS under the Centers for Disease Control and Prevention (CDC) is responsible for the development and maintenance of ICD-10-CM.

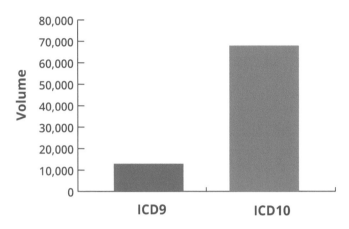

ICD-10 should produce a richer body of diagnosis and procedure data to help provide better trend analysis, a more detailed understanding of costs, and an ability to understand the effectiveness of managing care across the continuum. However, the conversion from ICD9 to ICD10 codes represents about a 300% increase in the number of codes that healthcare organizations will have to manage.

Structure & Terminology

The ICD-10 code sets are not a simple update of the ICD-9 code set, but show fundamental changes in structure and concepts that make them very different from ICD-9. It is not possible to convert ICD-9 data sets into ICD-10 data sets or vice versa. The table below compares the two data sets.

The ICD is updated and maintained by the **World Health Organization**.

27

ICD-9	ICD-10
3-5 characters in length	3-7 characters in length
Approximately 13,000 codes	Approximately 68,000 available codes
First digit may be alpha (E or V) or numeric; digits 2-5 are numeric	Digit 1 is alpha; digits 2 and 3 are numeric; digits 4-7 are alpha or numeric
Limited space for adding new codes	Flexible for adding new codes
Lacks detail	Very specific
Lacks laterality	Has laterality (i.e., codes identifying right vs. left)
ICD-9 Example: 3924, Aorta-renal Bypass	ICD-10 Example: 04104J3, Bypass Abdominal Aorta to Right Renal Artery with Synthetic Substitute, Percutaneous Endoscopic Approach

Logical Observation Identifiers Names and Codes (LOINC®)

Logical Observation Identifiers Names and Codes (LOINC®) is a universal code system that provides a definitive standard for identifying laboratory and clinical observations in electronic reports, thereby facilitating the exchange and pooling of results for clinical care, outcomes management, and research. LOINC was developed by the Regenstrief Institute, an internationally respected non-profit medical research organization associated with Indiana University. Regenstrief and the LOINC committee maintain this free and open system, and update it biannually, in June and December.

System Evolution

1994   Regenstrief investigators used their experience with electronic medical records to develop the Indiana Network for Patient Care, the nation's first citywide health information exchange. When confronted with difficulties in interpreting clinical content from various member institutions because each used a different code for the same test or observation, Regenstrief saw the need for a lingua franca, and LOINC was born. The initial release in 1995 had identifiers and names for about 6,000 laboratory test results.

2003   The U.S. Department of Health and Human Services (HHS) announced the first set of uniform standards for the electronic exchange of clinical health information across different sections of the federal government by adopting LOINC codes to standardize the electronic exchange of clinical laboratory results.

More than **20,000 people** in **150 countries** use LOINC to enable exchange and aggregation of electronic health data from many independent systems.

2005   HHS proposed the adoption of standards for claims attachments, which is information that providers attach to support claims for reimbursement. The proposal specified the use of Health Level Seven (HL7) messaging to transmit laboratory and clinical data. HHS adopted LOINC as the new HIPAA code set for these observations.

2012   The number of LOINC users grew to more than 14,500, in 145 countries, with over 58,000 observations.

Structure & Terminology

Each record in the LOINC database identifies a clinical observation with a code and formal name. For each observation, the database includes a sequentially assigned code (format: nnnnnn-n) with the last being a check digit, preceded by a hyphen to detect common typographic errors during manual entry. Besides the code, there are a long formal name, a "short" 30-character name, and synonyms. Each database record includes six attributes for the unique specification of each identified single test, observation, or measurement with this layout:

<component/analyte>:<kind of property>:<time aspect>:<system type>:<scale>:<method>

"Component|Analyte" is what is measured, evaluated, or observed, such as pain or potassium. "Property" means a characteristic of what is measured, such as length, mass, or temperature. "Time" is the interval over which the measurement is made. "System" is the context or specimen type, such as blood, urine, or patient. "Scale" can be quantitative, ordinal, nominal, or narrative. "Method" means what is used to describe the measurement or observation.

The LOINC database comes with a free mapping program called Regenstrief LOINC Mapping Assistant (RELMA) to support the mapping of local test codes to LOINC codes, and to facilitate browsing of LOINC results.

MEDCIN®

MEDCIN® is a proprietary medical vocabulary used as a clinical database engine during documentation by healthcare providers at the point of patient care. It is at present one of the largest numerically codified point-of-care medical terminologies in the world. MEDCIN® was developed and is maintained by Medicomp Systems, Inc., a company dedicated to the development of point-of-care tools for electronic health records. The vocabulary is updated quarterly.

System Evolution

1978   Peter S. Goltra, an electrical engineer and one of the founders of Medicomp Systems, Inc., determined to improve healthcare delivery after his father was diagnosed with ALS. Shocked that physicians could not find charts, or that records were incomplete, and that there were no standards governing the process of gathering, describing, and recording patient data, Mr. Goltra began a 30-year crusade to build a better system. He is now widely seen as a visionary in the field of medical informatics and a driving force in the mutually supportive blending of medicine and technology. He has collaborated closely with physicians from Cornell, Harvard, and Johns Hopkins Universities.

2005   First year of a multi-year plan to roll out MEDCIN® with the U.S. Department of Defense's electronic medical record system. The DOD joined a list of other high-profile MEDCIN® users, among them Epic Systems, Allscripts Healthcare Solutions, and WebMD.

MEDCIN contains **more than 280,000** clinical data elements encompassing symptoms, history, physical examination, tests, diagnoses, and therapies.

Structure & Terminology

MEDCIN® combines a database of over 280,000 clinical data elements with methods for presenting and documenting relevant symptoms, history, physical examinations, tests, diagnoses, and therapies related to any patient presentation, with the capability to cross-map to leading codification systems such as Systematized Nomenclature of Medicine—Clinical Terms (SNOMED CT), Current Procedural Terminology (CPT), International Classification of Diseases (ICD), Diagnostic and Statistical Manual of Mental Disorders (DSM), Logical Observation Identifiers, Names and Codes (LOINC), and the drug terminology database RxNorm.

Embedding MEDCIN in electronic health record systems allows the production of structured and numerically codified patient information, making interoperability easier and smoother. Such structuring permits aggregation, analysis, and mining of clinical and practice-management data related to a disease, a patient, or a population.

Medical Dictionary for Regulatory Activities (MedDRA®)

The Medical Dictionary for Regulatory Activities (MedDRA®) is a logical, international medical terminology used to classify adverse-event data associated with the use of biopharmaceuticals or medical products. MedDRA was developed under the auspices of the International Conference on Harmonization (ICH) and is a registered trademark of the International Federation of Pharmaceutical Manufacturers and Associations (IFPMA) acting as trustee for the ICH Steering Committee. MedDRA is managed by the Maintenance and Support Services Organization (MSSO), which releases annual updates in March and September.

System Evolution

1989
The United Kingdom Medicines Control Agency (MCA) identified the need for a single medical terminology for drug regulation to support its new computer database.

1993-1994
The MEDDRA Working Party enhanced the UK MCA's medical terminology to produce MEDDRA Version 1.0.

1997-1999
MedDRA Version 2.0 was chosen as the implementable version of the terminology at the ICH conference, and released two years later. A change in name and a modified acronym were agreed upon at this meeting. Hence, MEDDRA is used for versions up to Version

MedDRA® is a logical, international medical terminology used to **classify adverse-event data** associated with the use of biopharmaceuticals or medical products.

1.5, while the implementable (Version 2.0) and later versions are known as the MedDRA terminology.

2000s   MedDRA is continuously enhanced to meet the evolving needs of regulators and the industry around the world, with the latest version being 15.

Structure & Terminology

MedDRA has a five-level hierarchical structure in which each level's terms are mapped to the level above them and finally to a system organ class. The structural elements of the MedDRA terminology are as follows:

> » System Organ Class (SOC): Highest level of the terminology; divided into 26 classes, according to anatomical or physiological system, etiology, or purpose.

> » High-Level Group Term (HLGT): Subordinate to SOC; superordinate descriptor for one or more HLT's organized into clinically relevant groups.

> » High-Level Term (HLT): Subordinate to HLGT; superordinate descriptor for one or more PT's.

> » Preferred Term (PT): Represents the concepts in MedDRA, each being a specific and unique medical concept.

> » Lowest-Level Terms (LLT): Lowest level of the terminology and entry terms related to a single PT as a synonym, lexical variant, or quasi-synonym. (Each PT has an LLT identical to it.)

Each MedDRA term is assigned an eight-digit identification code without taxonomic meaning to facilitate electronic transmission. Additionally, the MedDRA dictionary includes Standardized MedDRA Queries (SMQ's), which were developed to facilitate retrieval of MedDRA-coded data as a first step in investigating drug safety issues in pharmacovigilance and clinical development.

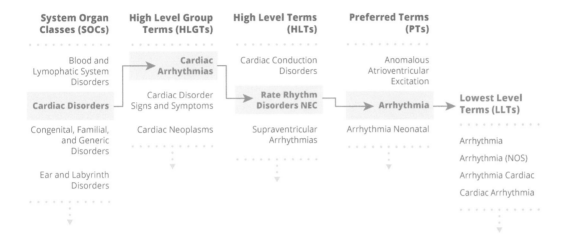

System Organ Classes (SOCs)	High Level Group Terms (HLGTs)	High Level Terms (HLTs)	Preferred Terms (PTs)	
Blood and Lymophatic System Disorders	**Cardiac Arrhythmias**	Cardiac Conduction Disorders	Anomalous Atrioventricular Excitation	
Cardiac Disorders	Cardiac Disorder Signs and Symptoms	**Rate Rhythm Disorders NEC**	**Arrhythmia**	**Lowest Level Terms (LLTs)**
Congenital, Familial, and Generic Disorders	Cardiac Neoplasms	Supraventricular Arrhythmias	Arrhythmia Neonatal	Arrhythmia
Ear and Labyrinth Disorders				Arrhythmia (NOS)
				Arrhythmia Cardiac
				Cardiac Arrhythmia

National Drug Codes (NDC)

N ational Drug Codes (NDC) are universal product identifiers for commercially available drug products intended for use in the United States. An NDC number uniquely identifies the manufacturer of a drug, the drug product, and its packaging size. The codes are created by the Food and Drug Administration (FDA), which maintains the NDC number and information submitted as part of the listing process in a database known as the Drug Registration and Listing System (DRLS). The published list is called the NDC Directory; it is updated quarterly.

NDC are used where the electronic exchange of information at the packaging level is desired, as in the retail pharmacy sector. However, NDC are also important for public health and safety. The FDA uses the Directory for, among other things, drug recalls and monitoring adverse drug events.

System Evolution

1969	The system was developed by the FDA as a directory for frequently-prescribed drugs for humans and as a method to identify drugs during commercial distribution.
1972	The Drug Listing Act dictated expansion of the NDC system to include over-the-counter and veterinary drugs for animals.
1990s	The Health Insurance Portability and Accountability Act (HIPAA) mandated the adoption of NDC as the standard medical data code set for reporting all drug transactions. This was a controversial decision, since drugs administered by physicians were billed using Healthcare Common Procedure Coding System (HCPCS) J-codes, not NDC.
2003	Under the Final Rule on Health Insurance Reform, the adoption of the NDC system for institutional and professional claims was repealed. The Rule retained

the use of NDC for all retail pharmacy transactions; however, since no standard medical code set was mandated for the other claims, trading partners could choose between NDC and HCPCS code sets.

Structure & Terminology

An NDC product identifier is comprised of three segments, separated by hyphens. The first segment, the labeler code, is assigned by the Food and Drug Administration. Its five digits identify the firm that manufactures, repackages, or distributes the drug. The second segment is the product code; it identifies the drug's strength, dosage medium, and formulation. The third segment is the package code, which identifies package sizes and types. Both the product and package codes are assigned by the firm identified in the first segment.

Under Section 510 of the Food, Drug and Cosmetic Act (FDCA, 1938), each drug product is assigned a unique 10-digit, three-segment number with one of the following configurations: 4-4-2, 5-3-2, or 5-4-1. Later, in order for consistency when the HIPAA standard called for an 11-digit NDC formatted as 5-4-2, other agencies used leading zeros for place values. To avoid confusion and preserve backward compatibility, the FDA stores complete NDC with an asterisk ["*"] placeholder instead of a leading zero.

The NDC system was developed by the U.S. Food and Drug Administration as a directory for **frequently-prescribed drugs** for humans and as a method to identify drugs during commercial distribution.

E-Prescribing

Pharmacies fill prescription medications using NDC codes. Ideally, prescribers order medications using RxNorm.

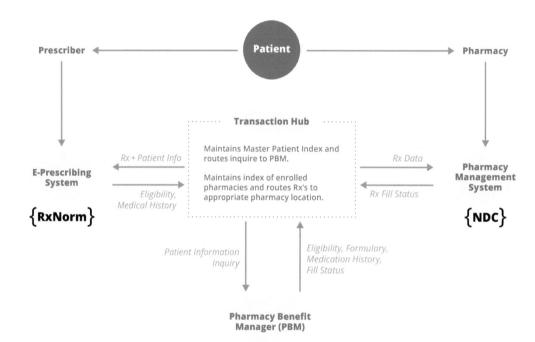

Resource-Based Relative Value Scale (RBRVS)

The Resource-Based Relative Value Scale (RBRVS) system determines healthcare reimbursements based on the relative value of the cost of resources to deliver a medical service. This mechanism assigns each procedure a relative value, adjusted by geographic region and multiplied by a fixed conversion factor, to determine the payment amount. Annual updates to the physician work-relative values are based on recommendations by a sub-group of the American Medical Association (AMA), the Specialty Society RVS Update Committee (RUC).

System Evolution

1980s   As a reaction to escalating healthcare expenditures, the U.S. Congress created the Physician Payment Review Commission (PPRC) to develop a new reimbursement model. It recommended a fundamental policy change in which the fee schedule was based on resource costs rather than on the previous standard, "customary, prevailing and reasonable" (CPR) charges.

1986   The Omnibus Budget Reconciliation Act (OBRA) mandated that the Department of Health and Human Services (HHS) develop an RBRVS to be submitted to Congress. The AMA's proposal generated antitrust concerns; to mitigate these, the Association accepted a proposal from Harvard to perform a national study. Research by principal investigator William Hsiao, Ph.D., and his colleagues resulted in the assignment of a numerical value or "weight," expressed in more than 7,500 Cur-

The Resource-Based Relative Value Scale (RBRVS) system determines **healthcare reimbursements** based on the relative value of the cost of resources to deliver a medical service.

rent Procedural Terminology (CPT) codes reflecting the complexity, time, training, and resources connected with a procedure or a service.

1989   Congress enacted the OBRA of 1989, mandating a Medicare Fee Schedule based on the RBRVS created from the Hsiao study, enhancing it with the inclusion of physician work, practice expense, and professional liability costs, as well as geographical adjustments. An annually updated conversion factor kept overall Medicare expenditures at the same level as in the prior CPR reimbursement model.

1991   The RUC was formed to make recommendations to the Centers for Medicare & Medicaid Services (CMS) on the relative values to be assigned to new or revised codes in the CPT book.

Structure & Terminology

The RBRVS breaks down the total cost of providing a particular physician service into three components (named "w", "pe," and "m") expressed in relative value units (RVU) where

>> **w** = the physician's own "work," which accounts on average for 52 percent of the total relative costs for each service;

>> **pe** = the physician's outlays for any practice expenses other than his or her own time (office space, supplies, clinical and administrative staff), which accounts for an average of 44 percent of the total relative cost of a service; and

>> **m** = professional liability insurance, accounting on average for 4 percent of total relative practice costs.

For a particular market area, each of these three cost components is adjusted by a Geographic Practice Cost Index (GPCI) that accounts for variations across market areas in the cost of living, the prices of non-physician practice resources, and malpractice premium rates. The sum of these geographically adjusted RVU's for a procedure constitutes the total RVU of that service.

The total RVU is converted into a dollar-value fee schedule by multiplying it by the annually adjusted conversion factor (CF) specified by statute. This factor is a dollar amount per RVU applied to all services in the relative value schedule. (The statute specifying the CF can be overridden by Congress when necessary.)

With all the above-defined elements in place, the formula looks like this:

Medicare Fee Schedule = [(RVUw x GPCIw) + (RVUpe x GPCIpe) + (RVUm x GPCIm)] x CF

The RUC Process

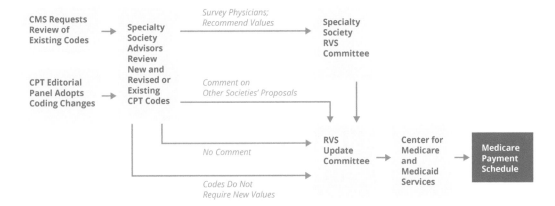

RxNorm

RxNorm is a standardized nomenclature for clinical drugs. The dataset has a normalized naming system for generic and branded drugs that supports semantic interoperation between drug terminologies and pharmacy knowledge base systems. The National Library of Medicine (NLM) produces RxNorm, updating it with newly-approved drug information every Wednesday. A new full RxNorm data set is released monthly.

System Evolution

2001   The NLM began an experiment in modeling clinical drugs in the Unified Medical Language System (UMLS) in the hopes that developing such a new method might lead to improved interoperability of drug terminology. This public-domain vocabulary project became known as the RxNorm Project.

2004   RxNorm was first released as an independent terminology, and established a monthly release schedule.

2010   The National Drug File Reference Terminology (NDF-RT) was integrated into RxNorm as a source vocabulary. NDF-RT is a resource developed by the Veterans Health Administration to add clinical properties (clinical use, mechanism of action, chemical structure, contraindication to use, possible interactions) to each drug name, allowing more sophisticated decision support.

2010   A Centers for Medicare & Medicaid Services (CMS)-commissioned RAND study recommended that RxNorm be adopted as the primary drug identifier in e-prescribing systems.

2012   CMS released Stage 2 Meaningful Use proposals, which stated that electronic health record vendors would have to begin incorporating standard clinical terminologies into their products, and include RxNorm for all medications.

Structure & Terminology

RxNorm is both a terminology in itself and a bridge between proprietary and open-source pharmaceutical resources. The NLM receives drug names from eleven data sources, analyzes and processes the data, and outputs the data into RxNorm files in a standard format. Like the Unified Medical Language System (UMLS) Metathesaurus, RxNorm is organized by concept. Each clinically distinct drug is grouped into a concept, and then assigned an RxNorm concept unique identifier (RXCUI), plus an RxNorm atom unique identifier (RXAUI) for each atom. Drugs whose names map to the same RXCUI are assumed to be the same drug—identical as to ingredients, strengths, and dose forms.

Next, strings with meaning, such as relationships and attributes from the source data, are attached to each concept. The eleven concept sources are: Gold Standard Drug Database, Medi-Span Master Drug Data Base, Medical Subject Headings (MeSH), Multum MediSource Lexicon, Micromedex Red Book, FDA National Drug Code Directory, FDA Structured Product Labels, FDB MedKnowledge, Veterans Health Administration National Drug File-Reference Terminology, SNOMED Clinical Terms, and Veterans Health Administration National Drug File. By providing links between and among these vocabularies, RxNorm can mediate messages between systems not using the same software and vocabulary, such as an electronic health record system and a proprietary pharmacy system.

The National Library of Medicine receives drug names from **eleven data sources**, analyzes and processes the data, and outputs the data into RxNorm files in a standard format.

43

RX NORM Overview

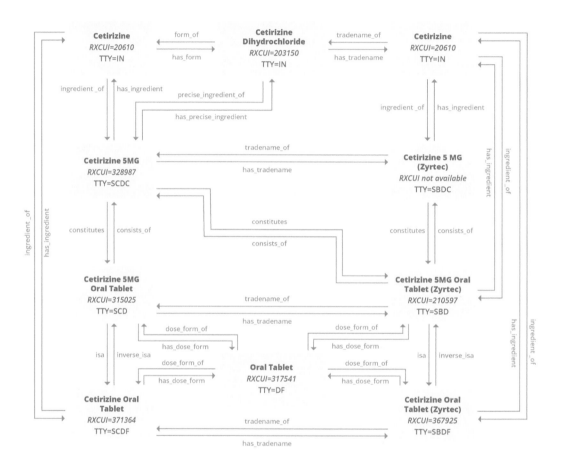

Standardized Nursing Languages (SNLs)

Standardized Nursing Languages (SNLs) are terminology sets used to describe the complex nursing process that consists of three principle components: assessment (diagnoses), problem-identification (interventions), and problem-management (outcomes). The evolution of SNL has spanned decades; currently, seven nursing-specific terminology sets have been approved by the American Nurses Association (ANA): NANDA International (NANDA-I), Nursing Interventions Classification (NIC), Nursing Outcomes Classification (NOC), the Clinical Care Classification System (CCC), the Omaha System, the Perioperative Nursing Data Set (PNDS), and International Classification for Nursing Practice (ICNP).

System Evolution

1973   Creation of the first standardized nursing terminology, named for the North American Nursing Diagnoses Association (NANDA), which devised it. This set of nursing diagnoses codifies clinical judgment about an individual, family, or community and its response to actual or potential health problems. Such an analysis differs from a medical diagnosis, as it deals with a disease or medical condition rather than a human response to symptoms or conditions. The Association's name later changed to NANDA-I to represent international participation; however the name of the dataset remained NANDA.

1975   The Division of Nursing of the U. S. Department of Health and Human Services funded the creation of the Omaha System, a practice and documentation standardized taxonomy

The development and use of a standardized language can help to reveal the impact of nursing care and **provide the consistency** required to compare interventions, outcomes and the quality of care across settings.

45

designed to assist in the documentation of care throughout the continuum of clinical care, including home health, ambulatory clinics, and hospital settings.

1988-1991	The CCC was developed from a research study conducted by Dr. Virginia K. Saba, EdD, RN, and a research team through a contract with the Health Care Financing Agency (HCFA), now Centers for Medicare and Medicaid Services (CMS). Originally called Saba's Home Health Care System, the CCC is designed specifically for electronic documentation of nursing care.
1992	Development of both the Nursing Interventions Classification (NIC) and the Nursing Outcomes Classification (NOC); these are maintained by the University of Iowa College of Nursing. They are comprehensive, research-based, standardized classifications of interventions and of outcomes, respectively.
1996	The International Council of Nurses (ICN) published an alpha version of the ICNP. The ANA, through a steering committee, has supported this international work when the existing systems had cultural translation problems. The World Health Organization (WHO) accepted ICNP within the WHO family of International Classifications to extend coverage of the domain of nursing practice as an essential and complementary part of professional health services.
1993-1999	The Association of periOperative Registered Nurses (AORN) Board of Directors recognized the need to develop a national computerized database specific to the field of peri-operative nursing to demonstrate to administrators and healthcare policy makers the patient problems that peri-operative nurses effectively manage. The PNDS is the first nursing terminology set developed by a specialty organization.

Structure & Terminology

Electronic documentation has accelerated the urgency of standardization, since the resulting heightened focus on quality outcomes necessitates a common language, to ensure that data extracted from different facilities reflects consistent information and results. Four of the seven terminology sets listed at the beginning of this essay include nursing diagnoses, interventions, and outcomes; conversely, a combination of NANDA-I, NIC and NOC equals their scope. Although not a nursing-specific terminology, The Systematized Nomenclature of

Medicine—Clinical Terms (SNOMED CT) allows for the use of multiple nursing language sets in a standardized format within an electronic health record. SNOMED CT also allows mapping by all of the nursing-specific terminologies. In terms of practice settings, NANDA, NIC, and NOC are frequently used in combination in the hospital, whereas the Omaha System and some of the other interface terminologies, such as the Perioperative Nursing Data Set or the Clinical Care Classifications, are used in community, home health, or other specialized clinical settings.

Sample Care Plan

NANDA Nursing Diagnosis

Risk for infection related to Immunosuppression secondary to chemotherapy, central venous catheter, chronic disease (ALL) and developmental level.

NOC Outcomes and Indicators

0702 Immune Status

Definition: Natural and acquired appropriately targeted resistance to internal and external antigens.

1 = *severely compromised thru*
5 = *not compromised*

Absolute WBC values WNL	1 2 3 4 5
Differential WBC values WNL	1 2 3 4 5
Skin integrity	1 2 3 4 5
Mucosa integrity	1 2 3 4 5
Body Temperature IER	1 2 3 4 5
Gastrointestinal function	1 2 3 4 5
Respiratory Function	1 2 3 4 5
Genitourinary Function	1 2 3 4 5
Recurrent infections	1 2 3 4 5
Weight loss	1 2 3 4 5

Etc....

NIC Intervention Label plus select nursing

6550 Infection Protection

Definition: Prevention and early detection of infection in a patient at risk

Activities:

Monitor for systemic and localized S&S of infection *(central line site check every 4 hours)*

Monitor WBC, and differential results *(q3rd day)*

Follow neutropenic precautions

Provide a private room

Limit number of visitors

Screen all visitors for communicable diseases

Maintain asepsis

Inspect skin and mucous membranes for redness, drainage *(every shift)*

Obtain cultures, as needed *(temp>38.3C q24h)*

Encourage fluid intake *(1300 cc/day, Pt likes 7up)*

Instruct pt to take antibiotic as prescribed *(ciprofloxin 500mg bid)*

Etc.....

Systematized Nomenclature of Medicine—Clinical Terms (SNOMED CT)

The Systematized Nomenclature of Medicine—Clinical Terms (SNOMED CT) is a controlled medical terminology developed specifically to facilitate the electronic storage and retrieval of clinical data. It is a multi-axial, hierarchical classification system where diseases can be defined by specific characteristics called axes. SNOMED CT is maintained by the International Heath Terminology Standards Development Organization (IHTSDO); English-language updates are released in January and July of each year. The National Library of Medicine (NLM) project "Unified Medical Language System (UMLS)" is the source for the United States license, and provides access at no charge.

System Evolution

1965   The Systematized Nomenclature of Pathology (SNOP) was developed for use by pathologists in codifying findings in their reports along four axes: topography, morphology, etiology, and function.

1970s   The Systematized Nomenclature of Human and Veterinary Medicine incorporated other clinical terms from all specialties, and expanded the axes to include disease, procedures, and occupations. These changes led SNOP to evolve into SNOMED, and later to SNOMED II.

1990s   SNOMED Version 3.x, also called SNOMED International, split the etiology axis into four, and a new axis for linking concepts was added. International Statistical Classification of Diseases (ICD) ICD-9-CM and Logical Observation Identifiers Names and Codes (LOINC) codes were mapped to SNOMED codes, making them suitable for use in any database application that coded patient information.

2000   Relational tables allowed for a new version, SNOMED RT, a concept-based reference terminology intended for implementation into electronic health records.

2002   The merger of SNOMED RT and Clinical Terms Version 3 (Read Codes) from the National Health Service in the United Kingdom created SNOMED CT.

2007   Responsibility for the ownership, maintenance, and distribution of SNOMED CT was transferred to IHTSDO, a nonprofit organization based in Denmark.

Structure & Terminology

SNOMED CT helps organize medical language into a structured framework. It is a collection of about 400,000 medical concepts, associated with about 800,000 descriptive terms for these concepts, ranged in a hierarchy (also known as a 'taxonomy') consisting of about 1,200,000 relations.

SNOMED CT is intended to be embedded into applications that record clinical information, such as the electronic health record. Recording information using SNOMED CT allows the information in the health record to be processed by computers. This in turn will enable: efficient searching of health records, retrieval of relevant clinical information, point-of-care decision support, automatic identification of patient risk factors, monitoring of response to treatment, monitoring of adverse reactions to treatment, long-term population disease or outcome analysis, and large populations of consistent data for medical research.

SNOMED is a collection of about **400,000 medical concepts**, associated with about 800,000 descriptive terms for these concepts, ranged in a taxonomy consisting of about 1,200,000 relations.

TNM (Tumor, Node, Metastasis) Classification

TNM (Tumor, Node, Metastasis) Classification is an anatomically based system for cancer staging. The three initials stand for the categories of cancer staging: the extent of the primary tumor is (T); the extent of spread to the lymph nodes is (N); and the presence of distant metastasis is (M). A number is added to each letter to indicate the size or extent of the primary tumor and the extent of cancer spread. In essence, the system is a shorthand notation for describing the extent of a particular malignant tumor.

The International Union Against Cancer, which is headquartered in Geneva, Switzerland (it is known by the initials of the main words of its title in French, L'Union internationale contre le cancer, or UICC) is responsible for the development and maintenance of TNM, with the continuing objective of achieving consensus in cancer classification.

System Evolution

1943-1952	Dr. Pierre Denoix developed the classification system at the Institut Gustave-Roussy in a suburb of Paris, France. Subsequently, the UICC established a Committee on Clinical Stage Classification under his leadership and continued to develop the TNM Classification.
1953	"Uniform Technique for a Clinical Classification by the TNM System" was published.
1960s-70s	Pocket guides (1st edition, 1968; 2nd editions, 1974) of the UICC TNM were published.
1980s	The International Federation of Gynaecology and Obstetrics (FIGO) developed the FIGO Classification for Gynaecological Malignancies and The American Joint

Committee for Cancer (AJCC) began publishing separate definitions of TNM categories. These parallel efforts were independent of the UICC TNM Classification.

1987   The unification of the UICC and American Joint Committee on Cancer (AJCC) for the 4th edition.

1990s   UICC TNM Classification of Malignant Tumours, 5th edition (1997)

2000s   UICC TNM Classification of Malignant Tumours, 6th edition (2002) and UICC TNM, 7th edition (2009)

Structure & Terminology

Primary Tumor (T)

» TX   Primary tumor cannot be evaluated

» T0   No evidence of primary tumor

» Tis   Carcinoma in situ (CIS); abnormal cells are present but have not spread to neighboring tissue

» T1, T2, T3, T4   Size and/or extent of the primary tumor

Regional Lymph Nodes (N)

» NX   Regional lymph nodes cannot be evaluated

» N0   No regional lymph node involvement

» N1, N2, N3   Involvement of regional lymph nodes (number of lymph nodes and/or extent of spread)

The three initials – TNM – stand for the **categories of cancer staging**: the extent of the primary tumor is (T); the extent of spread to the lymph nodes is (N); and the presence of distant metastasis is (M).

51

Distant Metastasis (M)

- » MX   Distant metastasis cannot be evaluated
- » M0   No distant metastasis
- » M1   Distant metastasis is present

Cancer staging can be divided into a clinical stage and a pathologic stage. In the TNM system, clinical stage and pathologic stage are denoted by a small "c" or "p" before the stage letter|number ID (e.g., cT3N1M0 or pT2N0).

In addition to c and p, there are other, optional descriptors (X, y, R, and r).

Unified Medical Language System (UMLS)

The Unified Medical Language System (UMLS) is comprised of centralized databases and associated software tools that assemble a comprehensive list of biomedical vocabularies and standards to enable interoperability between computer systems, including those storing electronic health records (EHR). The UMLS was initiated by the National Library of Medicine (NLM) and is maintained by a multidisciplinary team with public funding. The sources are updated semiannually in April and November, and can be used free of charge; however, they require a license agreement.

System Evolution

1986   Donald A. B. Lindberg, M.D., Director of the NLM, started a long-term research and development effort to meet an anticipated need for "intellectual middleware" to facilitate the development of advanced information systems that could retrieve and integrate information from a variety of disparate sources.

1990   Present. The NLM has issued annual editions of UMLS Knowledge Sources and associated lexical programs.

Structure & Terminology

The UMLS Knowledge Sources (databases) and related lexical programs (software tools) are accessible via the UMLS web-based Knowledge Source Server (UMLSKS), and are designed primarily for use by system developers or as reference tools for database builders and other informatics professionals. The system's three main knowledge components are:

One powerful use of the UMLS is linking health information, medical terms, drug names, and billing codes across **different computer systems**.

» The Metathesaurus® of medical concepts drawn from established vocabularies such as Systematized Nomenclature of Medicine (SNOMED), Current Procedural Terminology (CPT), Logical Observation Identifiers Names and Codes (LOINC), International Statistical Classification of Diseases (ICD), and RxNorm; the core database for UMLS. Each concept has specific attributes defining its meaning and is linked to the corresponding concept names in the various source vocabularies. There are over one million biomedical concepts and five million concept names with numerous relationships represented; for instance, hierarchical ones such as "is a" for subclasses, "is part of" for subunits, and "is caused by" for associative relationships. Each concept has a permanent Concept Unique Identifier (CUI) to which many individual source vocabularies are linked.

» The Semantic Network, a catalog of broad categories (semantic types) and their relationships (semantic relations) for all concepts represented in the Metathesaurus. Each concept in the Metathesaurus is assigned one or more of the 133 existing semantic types, which are linked with one another through one of the 54 semantic relationships. The semantic types are the nodes in the Network, and the relationships between them are the links. The major semantic types are organisms, anatomical structures, biologic function, chemicals, events, physical objects, and concepts or ideas.

» The Specialist Lexicon, which contains syntactic (describes how words are put together to create meaning), morphological (defines form and structure), and orthographic (refers to spelling) information for biomedical and common words in the English language. The Lexicon and its associated lexical resources are used to generate the indexes to the Metathesaurus and also have wide applicability in Natural Language Processing (NLP) applications.

Universal Medical Device Nomenclature System (UMDNS)

The Universal Medical Device Nomenclature System™ (UMDNS) is a standard international nomenclature and computer coding system for medical devices. UMDNS is owned and copyright by the Emergency Care Research Institute (ECRI), an independent nonprofit research organization devoted to applied research in healthcare, which updated it annually. Licenses may be purchased through the Institute. Nonprofit organizations are permitted to use this database free of charge.

System Evolution

1968	The ECRI formally began operation, focusing on research in emergency medicine, resuscitation, and related biomedical engineering studies. The Institute's first evaluation of 18 brands of manually operated resuscitators found nine to be ineffective. It responded to this discovery by founding ECRI as an independent evaluator and provider of medical-device-related information and guidance.
1971	The first version of the Universal Medical Device Nomenclature System was developed.
1997	ECRI Institute and the Center for Devices and Radiological Health of the U.S. Food and Drug

The UMDNS is a formal, hierarchical system that contains more than 26,000 medical device terms and 9,110 unique medical device concepts and definitions (preferred terms), along with **17,036 entry terms** to facilitate classifying of biomedical information.

Administration (FDA) agreed to mesh and standardize the UMDNS and the FDA's device-classification system.

2010   An ECRI Institute press release stated that the UMDNS contained 24,544 terms covering the entirety of medical devices and equipment used for modern health-care delivery, including information systems, software, in vitro diagnostics, molecular and genetic tests, capital equipment, implantable devices, assistive devices, and consumables.

Structure & Terminology

The UMDNS is a formal, hierarchical system that contains more than 26,000 medical device terms and 9,110   unique medical device concepts and definitions (preferred terms), along with 17,036 entry terms to facilitate classifying of biomedical information. A unique 5-digit numeric code|identifier corresponds to each preferred term.

For example:

>>   12912 Pacemaker, Cardiac, External Invasive

>>   16777 Catheters, Cardiac Balloon, Pulmonary Artery

>>   16488 Blood Glucose Monitors, Portable

>>   18504 Defibrillator|Cardioverter|Pacemakers, Implantable

>>   17577 Testers, Implantable Defibrillator|Cardioverter

The purpose of the UMDNS is to facilitate identifying, processing, filing, storing, retrieving, transferring, and communicating data about medical devices. The nomenclature is used in applications ranging from hospital inventory and work-order controls to national agency medical device regulatory systems, and from e-commerce and procurement to medical device databases. The U.S. National Library of Medicine incorporates the UMDNS into its Unified Medical Language System (UMLS) and the Institute of Medicine's Committee on Data Standards for Patient Safety has recommended the UMDNS as one of the core terminologies for electronic health records (EHR) Consistent device nomenclature supports quality, safety, and efficiency improvements such as enabling reporting from specialist EHRs to device registries (knee replacements, pacemakers, etc.); integrating home monitoring devices into EHRs; and enabling reporting of adverse events to MedWatch from EHRs.

The UMDNS is one of two international nomenclatures; the other is the Global Medical Device Nomenclature .

Select
Databases

Introduction: Select Databases

This section of the book contains compact descriptions, with histories, structures, and features, of healthcare databases selected for their interest and importance. We chose some because they are required for accreditation to provide certain services (Trauma, Bariatric, Cardiac), others because they document variations in healthcare delivery and in doing so have a significant effect on the shaping health policy (The Dartmouth Atlas of Health Care).

Like classification systems, these databases have evolved—in some ways quite significantly—in both design and the way they are used. Sometimes changing database structure and utilization mesh well with changes in the field; in many cases, they do not. For example, no matter how creative we are in using administrative (billing) databases, we will never be able to gain the depth of insight from them about the quality or outcomes of medical care that a well-defined and well-managed clinical quality-and-outcome database can offer.

We have tried to give you as much information as possible—in a concise and accessible format—about the most significant, widely used, and influential databases in healthcare research and design: where they come from, how they've changed, why they're still useful and effective today. Even with everything we've found, organized, updated, and presented, however, we have surely left some things out. Got a database you find crucial, but that we somehow missed? Please let us know. Our efforts to make this section and this book as complete and helpful as possible are ongoing, so we would love to hear from you.

Bariatric Outcomes Longitudinal Database (BOLD™)

The Bariatric Outcomes Longitudinal Database (BOLD™) is a proprietary outcomes database, established to assess the mid- and long-term outcomes of bariatric surgeries, and to analyze the relationship between these outcomes and (1) patient demographics and co-morbidities,(2) clinical and surgical characteristics, and (3) operative care and treatment. The data collected in BOLD is used to help ensure provider compliance with program requirements, and to develop general knowledge about best bariatric surgery practices. Although participation in the BOLD database is voluntary, it fulfills regulators' and third-party payers' requirements for credentialing and reimbursement for bariatric surgery. This comprehensive repository of bariatric surgery patient information is managed by the Surgical Review Corporation (SRC), an independent organization governed by industry stakeholders.

System Evolution

2003	The American Society for Metabolic and Bariatric Surgery (ASMBS) founded SRC and the Bariatric Surgery Centers of Excellence® (BSCOE) to address concerns about patient safety.
2007	The SRC developed the Bariatric Outcomes Database (BOLD) to accelerate development of clinical pathways and research for obese and diabetic populations.
2010	The SRC announced that the database now exceeded 250,000 patients, with an average accrual rate of 12,000 patients per month, making it the world's largest repository dedicated to the bariatric and metabolic surgical specialty.

2012   ASMBS and the SRC agreed to transfer administration of the Bariatric Surgery Center of Excellence (BSCOE) program to the ASMBS. The American College of Surgeons (ACS) and the American Society for Metabolic and Bariatric Surgery (ASMBS) announced plans to combine their respective national bariatric surgery accreditation programs into a single unified program to achieve one national accreditation standard for bariatric surgery centers. The 458 accredited and 200 provisional programs of the ASMBS BSCOE program joined the programs in the ACS BSCN to form the Metabolic and Bariatric Surgery Accreditation and Quality Improvement Program (MBS AQIP).

April 2012   All accredited programs began to report to the ACS BSCN data registry, labeled as a second-generation database.

Structure & Terminology

Patient data is collected for all phases of bariatric surgical care, including demographics, comorbidities, medications, surgical procedure type, weight loss and maintenance, adverse events, and outcomes. The data are self-reported; some are verified by on-site inspections. Surgical interventions covered in the registry include gastric banding, Roux-en-Y gastric bypass, sleeve gastrectomy, and biliopancreatic diversion with duodenal switch. The database provides a unique platform for evidence-based medicine, tracking complications, and improvement or resolution of comorbidities in an effort to develop risk-stratification guidelines that will promote improved patient care and outcomes. Researchers, payors, government, and other stakeholders interested in bariatric and metabolic surgery are strongly encouraged to use BOLD data, as doing so will help the bariatric community recognize trends, predict outcomes, develop global benchmarks, choose the right operation for each patient, improve the patient experience, and establish criteria for best practices.

In 2012, the American College of Surgeons (ACS) and the American Society for Metabolic and Bariatric Surgery (ASMBS) announced plans to combine their respective national bariatric surgery accreditation programs into a **single unified program** to achieve one national accreditation standard for bariatric surgery centers.

63

Cancer Registries

A cancer registry is an organized information system for the collection, storage, analysis, and interpretation of data on persons with the diagnosis of a malignant or neoplastic disease (cancer). Cancer registries are a primary source for unbiased population-based case control studies, the end points for cohort studies and clinical trials, and the beginning point for survival analysis. The data are collected by trained specialists, known as cancer registrars, who are represented by the National Cancer Registrars Association (NCRA). The primary focus of this not-for-profit association is leadership and certification for these cancer registry professionals. The U.S. Centers for Disease Control and Prevention (CDC) has established national standards to ensure the quality of cancer registry data.

System Evolution

1926   In the U.S., a limited type of bone sarcoma registry was established by Dr. Ernest Codman at Massachusetts General Hospital. The first fully-functioning hospital registry was at Yale-New Haven Hospital in Connecticut.

1935/1946   The first two central cancer registries were established, in Connecticut and California.

1956   The American College of Surgeons began to require the presence of a cancer registry as a pre-requisite for approved cancer programs.

1971   The National Cancer Act (centerpiece of "The War on Cancer") mandated that cancer-care facilities collect, analyze, and disseminate data for use in the prevention and treatment of cancer, and gave unique authority to the National Cancer Institute (NCI) to prepare and submit an additional annual budget (the "NCI Professional Judgment Budget") proposal directly to the president. The NCI is a component of the National Institutes of Health (NIH) and is the U.S. federal government's principal agency for cancer research and training.

1973   The Surveillance, Epidemiology, and End Results (SEER) Program of NCI established the first National Cancer Registry.

1992   The Cancer Registries Amendment Act, U.S. Public Law 102-515, established the National Program of Cancer Registries (NPCR). This program, administered by the CDC, provides support for states and territories to maintain registries that provide high-quality cancer data.

1993   State laws made cancer a reportable disease.

2003   The Cancer Biomedical Informatics Grid (caBIG) was created by NCI as an open-source cancer-based biomedical informatics network to enable cancer researchers to share tools, data, applications, and technologies to address the needs of NCI-based clinical trials and research.

2013   NCI has undertaken a thorough reassessment of the Cancer Biomedical Informatics Grid (caBIG) program and announced the launch of its replacement, the National Cancer Informatics Program (NCIP), intended to leverage the investments made in, and lessons learned from, caBIG.

Structure & Terminology

Cancer registries are of three general types: central registries, which are population-based entities that maintain data within certain geographical areas; healthcare institution registries, which are hospital-based, and maintain data on all patients diagnosed and|or treated at their facilities; and special-purpose registries that maintain data on a particular type of cancer, such the Gilda Radner Familial Ovarian Cancer Registry or the Central Brain Tumor Registry of the United States (CBTRUS).

Information maintained in the cancer registry includes:

Cancer data form much of the **body of knowledge** used by researchers, epidemiologist, public health officials and clinicians to understand, plan for and improve the quality of care for cancer patients.

» Demographic Information: age, gender, race|ethnicity, birthplace, residence

» Medical History: physical findings, screening information, occupation, prior incidence of cancer

» Diagnostic Findings: types, dates, and results of procedures used to diagnose cancer

» Cancer Information: primary site, cell type, and extent of disease

» Cancer Therapy: surgery, radiation therapy, chemotherapy, hormone, immunotherapy

» Follow-up: annual information on treatment, recurrence, and patient status is updated to maintain accurate surveillance information

The data are used to evaluate patient outcomes and quality of life; provide follow-up information; calculate survival rates; analyze referral patterns; allocate resources at regional or state levels; report cancer incidence as required by state law; and evaluate efficacy of treatment modalities.

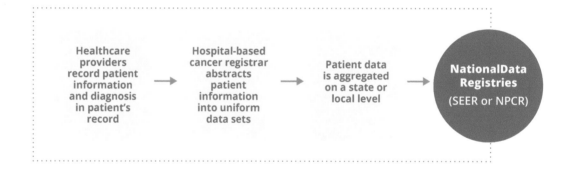

Centers for Medicare & Medicaid Services (CMS) Core Measures

ore Measures describe the basic care that should be provided to patients in hospitals, centered on evidence-based medicine research. Given that all stakeholders agree that it is reasonable to expect every patient with a particular diagnosis to receive the baseline (core) care established through research, United States healthcare providers are required to report their adherence to these measures to various governmental and independent regulatory agencies. In order to make data collection as streamlined, non-duplicative, and effective as possible, the Centers for Medicare & Medicaid Services (CMS) and the Joint Commission on Accreditation of Healthcare Organizations (JCAHO, commonly the Joint Commission, JC) have worked to align their versions of these measures so that they are identical, creating one common set of measure specifications, published and continually updated as The Specifications Manual for National Hospital Inpatient Quality Measures ("Specifications Manual"). These collaborative efforts are necessary because the CMS monitors a subset (Medicare patients only) of the JC data.

System Evolution

1982   The CMS Utilization and Quality Control Peer Review Organization (PRO) Program was shaped by the Social Security Act to improve quality and efficiency of services delivered to Medicare beneficiaries.

1987   The Joint Commission announced its "Agenda for Change," a plan designed to modernize the

Core Measures set national standards of care, and are a way to **compare the quality** of care that hospitals give.

accreditation process and pave the way for eventual introduction of standardized core performance measures.

Early 1990s The PRO Program evolved into CMS' Quality Improvement Organization (QIO) Program, a national infrastructure for healthcare measurement, reporting, and improvement.

1999 The JC decided on four initial core measurement areas for hospitals: acute myocardial infarction (AMI), heart failure (HF), pneumonia (PN), and pregnancy and related conditions (PR). The name ORYX® was chosen for the JC initiative that integrates outcomes and performance measurement data into the accreditation process.

2003 The CMS and the JC worked to align common-measure specifications for the QIO contracts and for JC-accredited hospitals: AMI, HF and PN measure sets. CMS also included Surgical Care Improvement Project (SCIP) measures.

2005 Section 5001(a) of the Deficit Reduction Act established a penalty for hospitals that did not submit data for all required quality measures to the QIO Clinical Data Warehouse: a reduction of 2% in their Medicare Annual Payment Update for the applicable fiscal year. This penalty system increased participation to 99%.

2008 Use of the Hospital Consumer Assessment of Healthcare Providers and Systems (HCAHPS) Survey was added to the requirements for participation in the CMS Hospital Quality Initiative to capture patient-satisfaction measurement. The program became known as Reporting Hospital Quality Data for Annual Payment Update (RHQDAPU).

2010 Readmissions for patients with CHF, AMI, and pneumonia were added as outcome results. CMS changed the name of the program to the Hospital Inpatient Quality Reporting (Hospital IQR) Program.

2012 The Hospital IQR Program measure set had by this date grown from a starter set of 10 to 72 quality measures with five focus areas: AMI, HF, PN, SCIP, and immunization coverage (the Global Immunization Measure Set).

2014   A new claim-based measure, Medicare Spending per Beneficiary, will by this year use claims data for hospital discharges for each episode, including all charges from 3 days prior to admission through 30 days post-hospital discharge. This would include Medicare A and B and any payments made by the beneficiary.

Structure & Terminology

Core Measures set national standards of care, and are a way to compare the quality of care that hospitals give. Each Core Measure reported represents the percentage of patients admitted with a specific diagnosis who receive the recommended care measures:

Number of patients receiving expected care ÷ Total number of patients with given diagnosis = %

Core Measures represent high-volume, high-cost diagnoses associated with an increased rate of morbidity or mortality, and are designed with the intent of doing the greatest good possible for the most people while supporting Value-Based Purchasing (VBP). (This new payment methodology rewards quality of care through payment incentives and transparency, replacing the fee-for-service payment model. VBP uses core clinical and patient satisfaction measures; facilities that maintain higher percentages of compliance with the core measures receive higher reimbursement from Medicare and other payers.)

69

Dartmouth Atlas Project (DAP)

The Dartmouth Atlas Project (DAP), also known as The Dartmouth Atlas of Health Care, maintains an online database of information on Medicare spending and use of selective services, providers, and facilities, by state, local, and regional market areas; by selected sub-populations of Medicare beneficiaries; and by providers. The interactive database also allows users to compare quality measures across hospitals. The database is a secondary data source, with the original data coming from The Centers for Medicare and Medicaid Services (CMS) administrative and claims data—Medicare Provider Analysis and Review (MEDPAR) files—and United States Census population data. The Dartmouth Institute for Health Policy and Clinical Practice administers this annually (or periodically, depending on indicator) updated database.

System Evolution

1973	First article on "Small Area Variation" published by John E. Wennberg, M.D., M.P.H., in the periodical Science.
1988	Having joined the Dartmouth faculty in 1980, Wennberg established The Center for the Evaluative Clinical Sciences (CECS) there.
1996	The Dartmouth Atlas of Health Care project was founded by Wennberg as part of the Dartmouth Institute for Health Policy and Clinical Practice. The first Dartmouth Atlas of Health Care was published.
2002	The MPH degree program in the Evaluative Clinical Sciences was established at the Dartmouth Institute.
2007	The CECS was reorganized as The Dartmouth Institute for Health Policy and Clinical Practice.
2008	Reporting of research data from the Dartmouth Atlas Project takes several forms, including periodic hard-bound volumes. In this year, the 20th such vol-

ume, The Dartmouth Atlas of Health Care: Tracking the Care of Patients with Chronic Illness appeared. Also in 2008, Wennberg received the Institute of Medicine's highest honor, the Lienhard Award, for his impact on the evolution of healthcare delivery in the United States.

Structure & Terminology

The DAP uses a population-based methodology called "small-area analysis," which focuses on the experience of a population living in a defined geographic area, or a population that uses a specific hospital. This type of data-collection and study is considered superior because healthcare usage in the United States is highly localized; that is, there is widespread variation in the way patients with chronic illness are treated medically. In some parts of the country, patients receive much more aggressive care—spending more days in hospitals and intensive care units and undergoing more tests and procedures, for example—than patients with the same diseases who live in communities where the pattern of practice is less aggressive.

DAP research supports a basic, two-part message: (1) there are unwarranted variations in healthcare use across regions in the United States; (2) more spending does not necessarily result in better healthcare quality, access to care, or health outcomes. Through its analyses, DAP suggests that improvements in both cost and quality can be achieved by supporting new models of payment that reward providers for improving quality, managing capacity wisely, and reducing unnecessary care.

DAP has conducted several state-based studies of all health insurance claims—both Medicare and commercial— that have shown that variations in resources and quality in the non-Medicare client group closely resemble those in the Medicare population, making the project's findings generalizable to the US population as a whole.

71

In 2008 John E. Wennberg, M.D., M.P.H., founder of the Dartmouth Atlas receives the Institute of Medicine's highest honor, the **Lienhard Award**, for "his impact on the evolution of health care delivery in the United States."

Data Elements for Emergency Department Systems (DEEDS)

Data Elements for Emergency Department Systems (DEEDS) is a set of recommendations published by the National Center for Injury Prevention and Control (NCIPC) of the Centers for Disease Control and Prevention (CDC) to adopt more uniform emergency-care data.

System Evolution

1994	A national conference on the status of emergency medicine, sponsored by the Josiah Macy, Jr., Foundation, spurred the development of DEEDS after participants acknowledged that shortcomings in available data limited their ability to answer many fundamental clinical, epidemiologic, and healthcare service questions about emergency department (ED) patients.
1994-1996	The CDC led a group of six professional associations and three federal agencies to co-sponsor and help plan and convene the National Workshop on Emergency Department Data. The January 1996 workshop (Atlanta GA) provided a public forum for review and discussion of an early draft of DEEDS.
1997	DEEDS Release 1.0 was finalized by a multi-disciplinary writing committee, then published and posted on the CDC website.

Structure & Terminology

DEEDS covers data elements in current clinical use; 156 elements are organized in the approximate chronological sequence of data acquisition during an emergency-department encounter. Eight sections include:

1) Patient Identification Data

2) Facility and Practitioner Identification Data

3) ED Payment Data

4) ED Arrival and First Assessment Data

5) ED History and Physical Examination Data

6) ED Procedure and Result Data

7) ED Medication Data

8) ED Disposition and Diagnosis Data

Hospital emergency departments in the United States serve a unique role in healthcare delivery, especially because they are the only institutional providers mandated by federal law to evaluate anyone seeking care. Because of the case mix and volume of patients treated, EDs are a rich source of data for public health surveillance, community risk-assessment, research, education, training, quality improvement, healthcare administration and finance, and other uses. DEEDS 1.0 specifications have been used for healthcare claims attachment specifications mandated by Health Insurance Portability and Accountability Act (HIPPA); emergency care terminology additions to the Logical Observations, Identifiers, Names, and Codes (LOINC) clinical vocabulary; and data definitions and terminology for public health surveillance initiatives. The data types and field lengths conform to Health Level Seven (HL7) specifications facilitating proposals to expand the scope of DEEDS to harmonize with disaster response systems and secondary data users such as the CDC and public health agencies.

73

Hospital emergency departments in the United States serve a unique role in healthcare delivery, especially because they are the only institutional providers mandated by federal law to **evaluate anyone** seeking care.

Healthcare Cost and Utilization Project (HCUP)

The Healthcare Cost and Utilization Project (HCUP, pronounced "H-cup") provides, in a uniform format, multi-state, administrative, population-based data that include information on both insured and uninsured patients. HCUP consists of a variety of databases, as well as related software tools and products developed through a federal-state-industry partnership and sponsored by the Agency for Healthcare Research and Quality (AHRQ). HCUP databases are "secondary data," assembling the data collection efforts of state data organizations, hospital associations, private data organizations, and the federal government (collectively known as HCUP Partners) to create a national information resource of patient-level healthcare data. The databases, released yearly, are accessible through HCUPnet, a free, on-line query system. Alternatively, many HCUP databases are available for purchase through the HCUP Central Distributor.

System Evolution

1988   Nationwide Inpatient Sample (NIS), a database of inpatient data from a group of over 1,000 hospitals, initiated the HCUP project.

1994   The Agency for Health Care Policy and Research (AHCPR, now AHRQ) developed HCUP Quality Indicators (QI's) in response to the increasing demand for information regarding the quality of healthcare. Today, the indicators are applied to HCUP hospital discharge data for several measures in the National Healthcare Quality Report (NHQR).

1995   Creation of State Inpatient Databases (SID), the second HCUP database set; they contain the universe of inpatient discharge abstracts from participating states.

1997   The Kids' In-patient Database (KID; a nationwide sample of pediatric in-patient discharges) and the State Ambulatory Surgery Databases (SASD; ambulatory care encounters from hospital-affiliated or freestanding ambulatory surgery sites) become the third and fourth additions to HCUP.

1999   State Emergency Department Databases (SEDD), sourced from hospital-affiliated emergency departments for visits that do not result in hospitalizations, marked HCUP's fifth database. In the same year, the HCUP central distributor was created by AHRQ with HCUP Partner organizations to prepare and distribute restricted-access, public-release versions of the databases for research outside of AHRQ on behalf of participating data organizations.

2006   The Nationwide Emergency Department Sample (NEDS), a database that yields national estimates of emergency department (ED) visits, became the fifth and most recent HCUP addition.

Structure & Terminology

HCUP, the largest collection of longitudinal hospital care data in the United States, includes selected data elements from inpatient and outpatient discharge records, including patient demographic, clinical, disposition and diagnostic|procedural information; hospital identification (ID); facility charges; and other facility information. The foundation of HCUP is billing data (UB-04, CMS 1500), plus any additional data elements from participating data organizations.

Each state forwards its data to AHRQ, which standardizes data to create a uniform format to facilitate both multistate and national-state comparisons and analyses. These databases are powerful resources that enable research on a broad range of health policy issues, including cost and quality of health services, medical practice patterns, access to healthcare programs, and outcomes of treatments at the national, state, and local market levels.

Healthcare Cost and Utilization Project (HCUP) is the largest collection of **longitudinal hospital care data** in the United States.

Healthcare Effectiveness Data and Information Set (HEDIS®)

ealthcare Effectiveness Data and Information Set (HEDIS®) is a set of performance measures designed to provide consumers and regulators with information to reliably compare competing managed-care health plans. HEDIS includes both clinical measures of care and measures of access to it; it is also used as a quality standard for healthcare organizations. The private, non-profit National Committee for Quality Assurance (NCQA), an organization dedicated to improving healthcare quality, developed and maintains the information; a committee oversees annual updates. HEDIS results are audited by an NCQA-approved firm, and are included in Quality Compass, an interactive, web-based comparison tool that allows users to view plan results and benchmark information.

System Evolution

1991	Version 1.0 of HEDIS, originally titled the Health Maintenance Organization (HMO) Employer Data and Information Set, was established.
1994	Version 2.0 was released as the Health Plan Employer Data and Information Set.
1997	Version 3.0 of HEDIS was released, and the NCQA announced that the acronym would stand for Healthcare Effectiveness Data and Information Set.
2000s	The HEDIS measure list began yearly updates, and was called "HEDIS [Current year]."
2006	HEDIS incorporated physician-level measures.

Structure & Terminology

HEDIS measures form a report card that evaluates a health plan's success in providing preventive care delivered by the physicians in a health plan's provider network. Over 90 percent of America's plans use the HEDIS tool to report more than 75 measures across 8 domains of care that address important health issues and serve as a component of the NCQA's accreditation process for these plans.

HEDIS measures include: counseling on smoking cessation; antidepressant medication management; breast health screening; cervical health screening; access for children and adolescents to primary care; immunization of children and adolescents; comprehensive diabetes care; management of hypertension; and prenatal and postpartum care, just to name a few. These measures are captured in three ways, each with its own methodology: Administrative, Hybrid, and Survey.

The Consumer Assessment of Healthcare Providers and Systems (CAHPS) survey is also included in HEDIS. The survey measures members' experiences with their healthcare in areas such as claims processing and getting needed care quickly, and asks them to rate their health plan on a scale of 1–10.

HEDIS is a surveillance asset designed to provide transparency to the healthcare system as part of healthcare reform, with the goal of simultaneously enhancing the experience of care, improving population health, and reducing per-capita costs.

HEDIS measures form a report card that evaluates a health plan's success in providing **preventive care** delivered by the physicians in a health plan's provider network.

Hospital Consumer Assessment of Healthcare Providers and Systems (HCAHPS)

The Hospital Consumer Assessment of Healthcare Providers and Systems (HCAHPS) Survey, also known as the CAHPS® Hospital Survey or Hospital CAHPS®, is a standardized survey instrument that measures and publicly reports patients' perspectives on hospital care. HCAHPS (pronounced "H-caps") enables valid comparisons to be made across all hospitals to support consumer choice. The Centers for Medicare & Medicaid Services (CMS) and the Agency for Healthcare Research and Quality (AHRQ; both agencies of the federal Department of Health and Human Services, HHS) created, and maintains, HCAHPS.

System Evolution

2002   CMS partnered with AHRQ to develop and test the HCAHPS survey.

2005   The HCAHPS survey was endorsed by the National Quality Forum. The federal Office of Management and Budget gave final approval for the national implementation of HCAHPS for public reporting purposes.

2006   CMS implemented the HCAHPS survey in October.

2007   Starting in July, the enactment of the Deficit Reduction Act of 2005 created a financial incentive for hospitals to participate in HCAHPS. Hospitals must collect and submit survey data in order to receive their full Inpatient Prospective Payment System (IPPS) annual payment update.

2012   The Patient Protection and Affordable Care Act of 2010 added HCAHPS to the measures used to calculate value-based incentive payments in the Hospital Value-Based Purchasing program, beginning with discharges in October 2012.

Structure & Terminology

The HCAHPS Survey asks discharged patients their opinions of numerous elements of their recent hospital stays. It covers critical aspects of the hospital experience (among others: communication with doctors, communication with nurses, responsiveness of hospital staff, cleanliness and quietness of the hospital environment, pain management, communication about medicines, discharge information, overall rating of hospital, and recommendation of hospital). In addition, sections of the survey help patients answer only appropriate questions; adjust for the mix of patients across hospitals; and support congressionally-mandated reports.

The survey can be implemented in four different modes: mail, telephone, mail with telephone follow-up, or active interactive voice recognition (IVR). The questionnaire, which takes on average about seven minutes to complete, is intended to provide meaningful comparisons of hospitals on topics that are important to consumers; create incentives for hospitals to improve quality of care; and enhance accountability in healthcare by increasing transparency of the quality of hospital care in return for public investment.

The HCAHPS Survey asks discharged patients their opinions of **27 elements** of their recent hospital stays. The results are publicly reported to support consumer choice and are used by Medicare to calculate value-based incentive payments.

Medicare Provider Analysis and Review (MedPAR)

The Medicare Provider Analysis and Review (MedPAR) file contains data from claims for services provided to beneficiaries admitted to Medicare-certified inpatient hospitals and Skilled Nursing Facilities (SNF). Each record in the MedPAR file represents an inpatient stay during the calendar year of the file and has information on diagnosis, procedure, charge, payment, provider, and patient for the claim. This collection of crucial information allows researchers to track inpatient history and patterns|outcomes of care over time. The Centers for Medicare and Medicaid Services (CMS) collects data for all U.S. hospital inpatient stays for Medicare beneficiaries and annually releases these data in the MedPAR file.

Data from the CMS are initiated through the Research Data Assistance Center (ResDAC), a consortium of faculty and staff from the University of Minnesota, Boston University, Dartmouth Medical School, and the Morehouse School of Medicine. ResDAC has a contract with CMS to provide free assistance to academic and non-profit researchers interested in using CMS (Medicare, Medicaid) data; however, there may be a fee connected with the data requested, depending on type and amount.

System Evolution

< 1995   MedPAR was created from claims from the Medicare quality assurance (MQA) system. At that time, a single MedPAR record represented an accumulation of adjustment claims.

Later   Inpatient and SNF claims from the National Claims History (NCH) file became the source of MedPAR. Further, each MedPAR record had evolved by this point to contain final-action claims data, with all adjustments resolved.

Structure & Terminology

The MedPAR File contains inpatient hospital and SNF final-action stay records for all Medicare beneficiaries. Each MedPAR record may represent one or multiple claim(s), depending on the length of a beneficiary's stay and the amount of services used throughout it. Useful data elements in the MedPAR file include: beneficiary demographic information, hospital provider number, length of stay, accommodation charges, diagnosis and procedure codes, and payment data.

The CMS offers three types of files to transmit its data. Research Identifiable Files (RIF) contain beneficiary-level protected health information. Requests for RIF data require a Data Use Agreement (DUA) and are reviewed by CMS's Privacy Board to ensure that the beneficiary's privacy is protected and the need for identifiable data is justified. Limited Data Set (LDS) files contain beneficiary-level protected health information; however, selected variables within the files are encrypted, blanked, or ranged. Public Use Files (PUF), also called Non-Identifiable Data Files, have been edited and stripped of all information that could be used to identify individuals. In general, PUF contain aggregate-level information on Medicare beneficiary or provider utilization.

Research and analysis using healthcare and financial data from MedPAR files has revealed interesting and inexplicable variations of resource utilization throughout the United States (see, for example, The Dartmouth Atlas), and has been a significant driving force behind healthcare reform in the U.S.

The Centers for Medicare and Medicaid Services (CMS) collects data for all **U.S. hospital inpatient stays** for Medicare beneficiaries and annually releases these data in the MedPAR file.

Minimum Data Set (MDS)

The Minimum Data Set (MDS) is a core set of screening, clinical, and functional status elements, including common definitions and coding categories, used by the Centers for Medicare and Medicaid Services (CMS) to support care management and reimbursement for long-term care residents. MDS is part of a Resident Assessment Instrument (RAI), an instrument developed by the CMS to standardize data collection from long-term care nursing facilities.

System Evolution

1986	The Institute of Medicine (IOM) study entitled Improving the "Quality of Care in Nursing Homes" led to the Omnibus Budget Reconciliation Act (OBRA) '87, which reformed nursing-home regulations. The IOM recommended that long-term care shift from structural evaluations of nursing homes to systematic, standardized assessments of residents' cognitive, functional, and emotional needs.
1987	OBRA called for the secretary of HHS to specify a minimum dataset of core elements for use in conducting comprehensive assessments of long-term care residents.
1990s	The Minimum Data Set and Resident Assessment Instrument were introduced in 1991; the former was revised in 1998, becoming MDS 2.0.
2000s	The CMS initiated a national project to create version 3.0 of the MDS, aimed at improving the clinical relevance and accuracy of MDS assessments and strengthening the voice of residents. A joint RAND|Harvard team led by Debra Saliba, M.D., M.P.H., revised the document with new emphasis on direct interviews of residents, and tested the new version from 2003 to 2008. The CMS implemented MDS 3.0 in 2010.

Structure & Terminology

MDS is the foundation of the comprehensive assessment of all residents of long-term care facilities certified to participate in Medicare or Medicaid. While it was originally designed as an assessment tool for identifying patient problems, its purpose has evolved. The data are used to create resident assessment protocols (RAPs), standardize communication, facilitate quality monitoring and improvement, and contribute to the design of the payment system. The daily rate paid to nursing homes is determined through the Medicare Prospective Payment System (PPS), which sets rates based on certain characteristics and the amount of resources used by residents. The grouping system is organized into Resource Utilization Groups (RUGs). The MDS is the primary driver of Medicare Part A reimbursement for skilled nursing facilities (SNFs) via the RUG system. When MDS 3.0 was introduced, so was RUG-IV. The RUG and other assessment information become part of the Universal Bill (UB-04) for claim billing.

The Minimum Data Set is the primary driver of Medicare Part A reimbursement for **skilled nursing facilities** (SNFs).

National Database of Nursing Quality Indicators (NDNQI®)

The National Database of Nursing Quality Indicators (NDNQI®) is a repository for nursing-sensitive indicators, reported at the nursing-unit level, designed to provide comparative information to hospitals for use in quality-improvement activities. Hospital site coordinators submit quarterly data by direct data entry to a secure website as part of a program of the American Nurses Association's National Center for Nursing Quality (ANA's NCNQI).

System Evolution

1994   The ANA launched the Safety & Quality Initiative to explore and identify the impact of healthcare restructuring on the safety and quality of patient care, particularly links between nursing care and patient outcomes.

1997   The ANA called for organizations to submit proposals to develop and maintain the NDNQI, then selected the Midwest Research Institute (MRI) and the University of Kansas School of Nursing to direct that program.

1998   NDNQI began accepting data from hospitals; three years later, it began charging for comparison reports.

2012   More than 1,800 U.S. hospitals had begun to participate in the database, with several NDNQI indicators endorsed through the National Quality Forum's (NQF) consensus measurement process.

Structure & Terminology

NDNQI's nursing-sensitive indicators built on and adapted the Donabedian conceptual framework. Avedis Donabedian, M.D., M.P.H., had collated the growing literature of health-services research, collecting the results in Evaluating the Quality of Medical Care (1966; the 2005 reprint by the Milbank Quarterly confirmed the relevance, timeliness, and continuing value of Donabedian's work). It emphasized the importance of evaluating health provision as to:

» structure (the supply, skill level, and education│certification of nursing staff)

» process (the nature and effectiveness of analysis tools for assessment, intervention, and RN job satisfaction)

» outcome (those patient outcomes determined to be nursing-sensitive—pressure ulcers, falls, IV infiltrations, or infections)

Besides providing comparative information, the database gathers, stores, and presents national data on the relationship between nurse staffing and patient outcomes. NDNQI reports identify quality improvement opportunities, satisfy regulatory reporting requirements, support RN recruitment and retention, promote patient development, and build quantitative foundations for policy research, budget planning, resource allocation, and staff education.

The NDNQI gathers, stores, and presents national data on the **relationship between nurse staffing and patient outcomes.**

National Hospital Ambulatory Medical Care Survey (NHAMCS)

The National Hospital Ambulatory Medical Care Survey (NHAMCS) is designed to collect data on the provision and use of ambulatory care services in hospital emergency and outpatient departments. The NHAMCS series gathers data from samples of patient records selected from emergency departments and outpatient departments of a national selection of hospitals that use a survey instrument known as the Patient Record Form. The Centers for Disease Control and Prevention, National Center for Health Statistics (CDC, NCHS), is the dataset owner of this annual survey. Its data, de-identified for protected health information, are available for downloading from the web at no cost.

System Evolution

1992   The NHAMCS was inaugurated to fill a gap in data on ambulatory medical care in the United States.

2006   A patient's drugs captured from the Patient Record Form began to be coded by their generic components and therapeutic classes using Lexicon Plus®, a proprietary drug database, replacing the previous, NCHS-developed drug-classification system.

2009   The data released began to include hospital-based ambulatory surgery centers.

2010   NHAMCS began to collect information from freestanding ambulatory surgery centers.

Structure & Terminology

The annually-released NHAMCS public-use dataset comprises two separate files: one for out-patient-department visits, the other for emergency-department visits. Each record in the file contains a complete description of the ambulatory care visit, based on information provided on the Patient Record. These data-collection forms vary slightly from year to year; however, the overall format of the survey has remained consistent.

The main focus of the survey is on the content of the individual visit: gathering clinician and institutional characteristics; patient details including demographic information and insurance status, vital statistics, reason for the visit, and diagnoses related to the visit; diagnostic and screening services and non-medication-based treatments ordered or provided; medications (including immunizations and other office-administered drugs) prescribed; and visit disposition. Participating physicians (and their patients) vary from year to year, prohibiting longitudinal follow-up, although the serial cross-sectional nature of the survey allows for tracking of trends over time.

Sampling is conducted using a multi-stage stratified probability approach; visit weights and clustering variables are available to convert survey data to nationally representative estimates of annual utilization of hospital outpatient departments or emergency departments in the United States. Diagnosis, cause of injury, and procedure data are coded using the International Classification of Diseases (ICD-9-CM). Reasons for visit are coded using internal systems developed by the NCHS.

The NHAMCS was inaugurated to fill a gap in data on **ambulatory medical care** in the United States.

87

National Hospital Care Survey (NHCS)

The National Hospital Care Survey (NHCS) replaces, as of 2011, the National Hospital Discharge Survey (NHDS). The NHCS integrates hospital inpatient data collected by NHDS with data collected by the National Hospital Ambulatory Medical Care Survey (NHAMCS); the latter includes emergency departments, outpatient departments, hospital-based ambulatory surgery locations, and free standing ambulatory surgery centers results. The NHCS has been redesigned to examine encounters of care across both inpatient and outpatient settings. It is sponsored by the Center for Disease Control's (CDC's) National Center for Health Statistics (NCHS), the nation's principal health statistics agency.

System Evolution

1960   The National Office of Vital Statistics was merged with the National Health Survey to establish the National Center for Health Statistics (NCHS), and four years later initiated the National Hospital Discharge Survey after a feasibility study by the University of Pittsburgh's School of Public Health.

1965-2010   The NHDS, a national probability survey designed to meet the need for information on characteristics of inpatients discharged from non-Federal short-stay hospitals in the United States, was conducted annually. The data it gathered covered both patient information (demographics, length of stay, diagnoses, procedures) and hospital characteristics (region, ownership, number of beds).

2011   NCHS replaced the NHDS with the NHCS.

2013   Ambulatory care data became part of the NHCS when the National Hospital Ambulatory Medical Care Survey (NHAMCS) was included. It added data on hospital

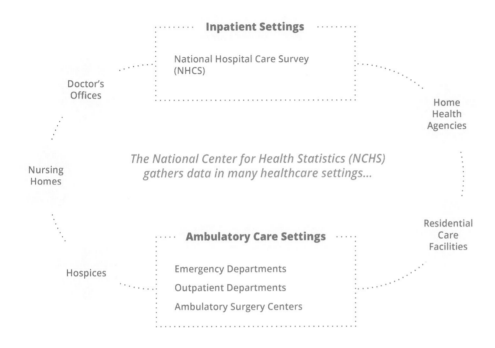

Inpatient Settings

National Hospital Care Survey (NHCS)

Doctor's Offices

Home Health Agencies

Nursing Homes

The National Center for Health Statistics (NCHS) gathers data in many healthcare settings...

Residential Care Facilities

Hospices

Ambulatory Care Settings

Emergency Departments

Outpatient Departments

Ambulatory Surgery Centers

89

characteristics, patient demographics (age, sex, race, ethnicity), and visit parameters (symptoms, complaints or other reasons for the visit; diagnoses; diagnostic and therapeutic services ordered or provided at the visit, including medications; expected sources of payment; visit disposition).

Structure & Terminology

Data for the inpatient component of the survey comes from Uniform Bill (UB-04) claims data and from chart abstraction for special studies. Ambulatory data is gathered through chart abstraction from the medical records. As hospitals adopt electronic health records, NCHS will accept electronic files from hospital medical records for all components of the survey.

NHCS provides nationally representative data on utilization of **hospital inpatient care**, as well as hospital ambulatory care.

NHCS provides nationally representative data on utilization of hospital inpatient care, as well as hospital ambulatory care. Patient-level identifiers are collected, allowing the information to be linked to episodes of care across hospital units as well as to other data sources, such as the National Death Index (NDI), to measure post-discharge mortality; and finally to Medicare and Medicaid claims databases [Medicare Provider Analysis and Review (MedPAR) and Medicaid Statistical Information System (MSIS), respectively] to obtain a wide-ranging view of patient care. NCHS compiles statistical information from the survey to help guide public health and health policy decisions, and provides data access to help answer key questions from healthcare professionals and researchers.

National Surgical Quality Improvement Program (NSQIP)

The National Surgical Quality Improvement Program (NSQIP) is a surgical outcomes database of the American College of Surgeons (ACS). The ACS NSQIP is the only nationally benchmarked, clinical, risk-adjusted, outcomes-based program to measure and improve care across the surgical specialties in private-sector hospitals. Hospitals enrolled in the ACS NSQIP have their data presented to them via comprehensive semiannual summaries and real-time, continuously updated, online benchmarking reports.

System Evolution

1985   The U. S. Congress established Public Law No. 99-166, a mandate to improve surgical outcomes among Veterans Administration (VA) hospitals. This law was designed to remedy an observed high rate of mortality and surgical complications. The effectiveness of this provision was unfortunately limited by the absence of a risk-adjusted database, and of reliable national averages for surgical outcomes.

1991-1993   The National VA Surgical Risk Study led to the creation of parameters of risk adjustment.

1994   The VA-NSQIP was created, allowing risk-adjusted comparison of the 133 VA hospitals and eventually reducing mortality by 27% and morbidity by 45%.

In 1994 the VA-NSQIP was created, allowing risk-adjusted comparison of the **133 VA hospitals** and eventually reducing mortality by 27% and morbidity by 45%.

1992-2002   The ACS, inspired by the VA-NSQIP's success, conducted a pilot study with seven private hospitals and 14 academic centers, validating the VA results.

2004   The ACS made participation in the NSQIP available to all private-sector hospitals in the United States.

2011   As of this year, over 300 hospitals were participating in NSQIP.

Structure & Terminology

ACS NSQIP collects data on over one hundred variables, including demographics, surgical profile, preoperative risk factors, intra-operative variables, and 30-day postoperative mortality and morbidity outcomes for patients undergoing major surgical procedures in both inpatient and outpatient hospital settings. The data are collected, validated, and submitted by a trained Surgical Clinical Reviewer (SCR) at each site. Each hospital submits an average of 1,600 major operations per year to the NSQIP database. Multiple categories of complications are reported; the variables are subjected to logistic regression to determine their ability to predict the risk of complications. Risk-adjusted outcomes are calculated using the patient variables submitted by each hospital. This risk adjustment allows unbiased comparison of results between hospitals of different sizes serving different patient populations.

ACS NSQIP collects clinical patient data (not insurance claim data) through chart abstraction that empowers surgeons and hospitals to compare their clinical outcomes to those of similar patients and hospitals and to identify opportunities to improve. The collected data is risk-adjusted, case-mix adjusted, and based on 30-day outcomes.

National Trauma Data Bank® (NTDB)

The National Trauma Data Bank® (NTDB) is the largest aggregation of U.S. / Canadian trauma-registry data ever assembled. The National Trauma Data Standard (NTDS; formerly known as the National Trauma Registry, NTR) is a dataset defining standardized data elements collected by the American College of Surgeons (ACS) within the NTDB. Each individual hospital trauma registry may also collect additional variables important to patient care on its own; however, the NTDS includes only core variables that would prove useful if aggregated on a national level. Data thus aggregated contribute to annual, hospital benchmark, and data-quality reports to inform the medical community, the public, and decision-makers about a wide variety of issues that characterize the current state of care for injured persons. The NTDB is a registered trademark of the ACS, which collaborates with Digital Innovation, Inc., on technical support for the NTDB Data Center.

System Evolution

1966 The Committees on Trauma and on Shock of the National Academy of Sciences, collaborating with the National Research Council, released the white paper "Accidental Death and Disability: The Neglected Disease of Modern Society." This was the first such paper to recognize the need for a trauma registry.

1983 The Major Trauma Outcome Study (MTOS), a retrospective study coordinated through the ACS Committee on Trauma, prefigured and probably led to the establishment of the NTDB.

In 2004 the NTDB reached the **one-million-records** mark, and began a project on data-element standardization.

93

1989	The NTDB was established with significant resources from the Board of Regents of the ACS.
1995	The ACS Committee on Trauma convened a consensus conference with trauma-registry program representatives to define NTDB data elements.
1997-1999	First call for NTDB data and data analysis 2001–Release of the first NTDB Annual Report
2004	The NTDB reached the one-million-records mark, and began a project on data-element standardization.
2005	The NTDB and the Centers for Disease Control and Prevention (CDC) collaborated on the National Sample Program (NSP), a national probability sample of 100 Level I and II trauma centers in the United States. The Program provides baseline estimates of trauma care to support trauma-care assessment, clinical outcomes research, and injury surveillance.
2006	The new data dictionary, the National Trauma Data Standard, was released.

Structure & Terminology

The Data Bank lists fifty-six data elements from ten information categories: patient demographics, injury, pre-hospital, emergency department, hospital procedure, diagnosis, injury severity, outcome, financial, and quality assurance. Every trauma center extracts these data elements from the patient's medical record and deposits its data into the bank. Data withdrawals from the bank are used to assess trauma systems and institutional performance, and for clinical and epidemiological research. The outcome most commonly studied in trauma populations is hospital mortality.

National Vital Statistics System (NVSS)

The National Vital Statistic System (NVSS) is a cooperative, decentralized system for inter-governmental data-sharing in the area of public health. Data from over six million vital event records (every birth, death, and fetal death record in the nation) are collected each year by 57 vital-registration jurisdictions that comprise each state, New York City, the District of Columbia, and five U.S. territories, and are sent to the Centers for Disease Control and Prevention's (CDC's) National Center for Health Statistics (NCHS) for processing and dissemination. From this trove, NCHS, the nation's principal health statistics agency, compiles information that guides public health and policy decisions through a cooperative arrangement with each jurisdiction.

System Evolution

Pre-1950   The birth of the NVSS system can be traced to the creation of the Bureau of the Census in 1902. Congress gave the bureau statutory authority to establish registration areas to produce nationally comparable vital statistics. In 1946, the bureau transferred its vital statistics responsibility to the National Office of Vital Statistics in the Public Health Service.

1960   The National Office of Vital Statistics merged with the National Health Survey to establish

Data from over **six million vital event records** (every birth, death, and fetal death record in the nation) are collected each year by 57 vital-registration jurisdictions that comprise each state, New York City, the District of Columbia, and five U.S. territories, and are sent to the Centers for Disease Control and Prevention's (CDC's) National Center for Health Statistics (NCHS) for processing and dissemination.

the NCHS, which became part of the CDC of the U.S. Department of Health and Human Services in 1987.

1981   The National Death Index (NDI), a supplementary data source, was established to aid researchers.

1994   A working group was formed by NCHS and state partners, represented by the National Association of Public Health Statistics and Information Systems (NAPH-SIS), to begin discussions of re-engineering the death-registration system using state-of-the-art technology.

2003   Revised U.S. Standard Certificates of Live Births and Deaths and the Fetal Death Report were developed.

Structure and Terminology

NCHS collaborates with NAPHSIS and the Social Security Administration to develop standards and efficient models for collecting information from a myriad of contributors—physicians, nurse-midwives, medical examiners, coroners, funeral directors, hospital and clinic directors, clerks, and temporary staff who complete the worksheets and certificates that eventually become data driving public health issues and policy decision-making. The NVSS includes several major electronic data files, each containing demographic and health information recorded on that file's particular events.

The natality file records birth data: mother's age, race, ethnicity, education, residence, marital status, month of pregnancy, month prenatal care began, tobacco use, and weight gain during pregnancy; and characteristics of the birth itself: birth weight, length of gestation, gender, whether a multiple birth occurred, method of delivery, and congenital anomalies.

The mortality file records death data variables: residence, place of occurrence, month of death, age, race, ethnicity, birthplace, gender, education, marital status, and underlying and multiple causes of death. The fetal death file includes data on all fetal deaths of twenty weeks' or more gestation and also includes the fetal or maternal conditions causing death.

NCHS works in partnership with the vital registration systems in each jurisdiction to produce critical information on such topics as teenage births and birth rates, prenatal care and birth weight, risk factors for adverse pregnancy outcomes, infant mortality rates, leading causes of death, and life expectancy. The data are used to track the impact of major policy initiatives including the Affordable Care Act and to identify disparities in health status and the use of health care by race|ethnicity, socio-economic status, and geographic region. Since September 11, 2001, it has been recognized that vital records office have, besides the civil registration of vital events and the collection of public health data, the crucial function of helping to ensure national security.

Outcome and Assessment Information Set (OASIS)

The Outcome and Assessment Information Set (OASIS) is part of a comprehensive assessment and reporting tool required for all adult home care patients receiving skilled care reimbursed by Medicare or Medicaid. This multi-purpose data set is used to produce quality reports for agencies and for public reporting on the Medicare Home Health Compare website. In addition to quality measurement, a subset of OASIS items is used to calculate payment algorithms under the Medicare Prospective Pay System (PPS). OASIS data are submitted by home health agencies to the States, and subsequently transmitted to the Centers for Medicare & Medicaid Services (CMS), which is responsible for maintaining the dataset.

System Evolution

1987   The Omnibus Budget Reconciliation Act mandated that Medicare monitor the quality of home healthcare and services with a "standardized, reproducible" assessment instrument and the following year, Health and Human Services (HHS) contracted with University of Colorado researchers and clinicians to develop such an instrument.

1994-1998 The first OASIS was published followed by years of refinement through several iterations of clinical and empirical research resulting in OASIS-A, then B, and finally OASIS B-1 in 1998.

1999-2000 The runaway home health expenditures that marked the mid-1990's provided the impetus for Congress to enact the home health provisions in the Balanced Budget Act (BBA) of 1997. Home Health PPS was implemented on October 1, 2000. Under PPS, a prospectively determined per-episode payment rate is case-mix adjusted using 80 mutually exclusive Home Health Resource Groups

(HHRGs). Each Medicare episode is classified into an HHRG using a subset of items from the Outcome and Assessment Information Set (OASIS) that was submitted to Medicare.

2008   Changes were made to the OASIS-B1 to reflect the new 2008 Home Health PPS, in which HHRG combinations increased from 80 to 153.

2010   OASIS-B1 is revised and renamed to OASIS-C. The OASIS-C includes process items that will support the public reporting of evidence-based practices and advances the standardization of many OASIS assessment items. The Minimum Data Set (MDS) and the Continuity Assessment Record Evaluation (CARE) instruments being developed for use across all post-acute care settings may signal an end to the need for OASIS in the future.

Structure & Terminology

OASIS data elements encompass a wide range of socio-demographic, environmental, health status, health service utilization, and functional status characteristics of adult patients, which are designed to enable systematic comparative measurement of home healthcare patient outcomes at two points in time. Each data element is referred to as "MOO" items, where M= Medicare and 00 = Numbers that identify the specific OASIS item. For example, under the Respiratory Status section of the assessment:

(M1410) Respiratory Treatments utilized at home (mark all that apply):

1)   Oxygen (intermittent or continuous)

2)   Ventilator (continually or at night)

3)   Continuous | Bi-level positive airway pressure

4)   None of the above

OASIS data are collected at start of care, on a 60-day follow-up cycle, and at discharge. The OASIS quality data submitted by home health agencies to state repositories

OASIS data is part of a comprehensive assessment for all **adult home care patients** who are receiving skilled care that is reimbursed by Medicare or Medicaid.

are stored in the Quality Improvement Evaluation System (QIES) database. To ease the cost burden of data submission, Home Assessment and Validation and Entry (HAVEN) data entry software is available free of charge from CMS.

PatientsLikeMe (PLM)

PatientsLikeMe (PLM) is a free, data-driven social networking health site offering a personalized research and peer-care platform where members share in-depth information on conditions, treatments, and outcomes. The site offers access to powerful tools (clinical assessment tests, algorithms) that can predict, based on the progression of the disease and other factors, how long someone is likely to live. PLM was developed by PatientsLikeMe, Inc., whose transparent business model collects and sells de-identified data to drug and medical-device companies for marketing and clinical research.

System Evolution

2004   MIT engineers Benjamin and James Heywood and Jeff Cole co-founded the company, inspired by the courage of their brother and friend Stephen Heywood in the face of Amyotrophic Lateral Sclerosis (ALS | Lou Gehrig's disease).

2006   Neuropsychologist Paul Wicks joined the company as the site launched, leading the transformation of PLM from an online outpost for ALS patients into a passionately engaged global community of people with more than 1,000 serious conditions, including cancer, multiple sclerosis, diabetes, and HIV | AIDS.

2009   PLM proved that self-reported data had real value in clinical research when it published a study in Nature Biotechnology arguing that lithium carbonate does not slow the progression of ALS. This article contradicted an earlier clinical study that had claimed to show promise in ALS treatment with the drug. In the same year, PLM moved toward more precise,

Historically, healthcare information has flowed from researchers and specialists, not from patients; however, new **social network platforms** are creating faster, more patient-centric information flows.

solid reporting as it began to code adverse drug events with the Medical Dictionary for Regulatory Activities (MedDRA), and set up a channel to submit this data to the U.S. Food and Drug Administration (FDA).

2011   PLM had grown into one of the leading user-reported medical sites (over 110,000 members; worldwide support for thousands of diseases). It allowed system subscribers visual access to a list of those trials on ClinicalTrials.gov that were tailored to their conditions and demographics.

Structure & Terminology

PLM contributes both to immediate empowerment (by helping patients improve their own care) and ongoing progress toward healing (by supporting the development of new therapies, in partnership with the industry, through the contribution of well-codified data). Members input real-world information on their conditions, treatment history, side effects, symptoms, quality of life, weights, lab values, and disease-specific functional scores. (They use, among others, the Revised ALS Functional Rating Scale (ALSFRS-R) and the Unified Parkinson's Disease Rating Scale (UPDRS-III). This ongoing data stream builds a detailed longitudinal record organized into charts and graphs that reveal useful insights and patterns.

Historically, healthcare information has flowed from researchers and specialists, not from patients; however, new social network platforms are creating faster, more patient-centric information flows. Establishing the right balance among patient, clinical, and research perspectives is central to integrating this complex data over multiple domains to uncover patterns and present new ideas on diagnosis and treatment. Many conditions affecting PLM members are treated with off-label therapies; ideally, the site will become a rich and productive source of evidence on these secondary uses, highlighting prime targets for traditional clinical trials that could lead to even more effective treatments. While not a replacement for the gold-standard, double-blind clinical trial, the platform can provide supplementary data to support effective decision-making in medicine and discovery.

Pediatric Quality Measures Program (PQMP)

The Pediatric Quality Measures Program (PQMP) is a federally mandated initiative drafted in response to a finding by the Institute of Medicine (IOM) that the United States, despite the presence of multiple datasets and measures, had no robust national information system to provide timely, comprehensive, and reliable indicators of health and healthcare quality for children. The goal of the Program is to strengthen and expand on existing pediatric quality measures and increase the portfolio of evidence-based, consensus-driven ones available to public and private purchasers of children's health care services, to providers, and to consumers. The PQMP is managed and run under the Children's Health Insurance Program Reauthorization Act (CHIPRA), part of national policy efforts underway to improve pediatric health care quality.

System Evolution

2009   Congress passed the CHIPRA, Public Law 111-3, which provided states with new funding and incentives to cover children through Medicaid and the Children's Health Insurance Program (CHIP). The law tasked the Secretary of Health and Human Services (HHS) with developing standards by which states could measure the quality of the care that children received. The Agency for Healthcare Research & Quality (AHRQ) and Centers for Medicare & Medicaid Services (CMS) partnered to implement selected provisions of the law, in two phases.

The goal of the Program is to strengthen and expand on existing pediatric quality measures and increase the portfolio of **evidence-based, consensus-driven** ones available to public and private purchasers of children's health care services, to providers, and to consumers.

2010   Phase I deadline for identification of initial core set of measures for voluntary use by Medicaid and CHIP programs.

2011   Phase II deadline for development of a Pediatric Quality Measures Program. AHRQ announced seven cooperative grant awards for the CHIPRA Pediatric Quality Measurement Program (PQMP) Centers of Excellence (CoE). Each CoE would comprise multiple entities with diverse expertise charged with seeking resolution of some of the most pressing issues in child health quality measurement.

2013   Posting of improved core sets of children's healthcare quality measures for voluntary use by State Medicaid and CHIP programs, private sector insurers, providers, and other stakeholders.

Structure & Terminology

The CHIPRA Pediatric Quality Measures Program requires measures that are evidence-based, understandable, equipped to identify disparities, and able to measure quality at the state, health-plan, and provider levels of aggregation. According to the IOM, PQMP structure must make better use of existing data, integrate different data sources and develop new ones, and devise collection methods for unique populations to meet these requirements. Existing administrative data comes from the Medicaid Statistical Information System (MSIS) for state-level Medicaid claims and encounter data, and from the Healthcare Effectiveness Data and Information System (HEDIS) for managed care beneficiary data. Current quality measures as well as administrative data can be found in population health surveys. The National Survey of Children's Health (NSCH) and the National Survey of Children with Special Health Care Needs (NS-CSHCN) touch on multiple, intersecting aspects of children's lives: physical and mental health, access to quality health care, and the child's family, neighborhood, and social context. The Data Resource Center for Child and Adolescent Health (DRC) makes survey data easily accessible to researchers and consumers.

The Patient Protection and Affordable Care Act (PPACA) of 2010 emphasized all populations of children, regardless of payer, hence the need for new sources of data to provide information on these. An overarching goal is expansion of all sources and linkage with other databases to build a national information system that can accurately report the quality of children's healthcare.

Prescription Drug Monitoring Programs (PDMPs)

Prescription Drug Monitoring Programs (PDMPs) are statewide electronic databases that gather information from pharmacies on dispensed prescriptions for controlled substances. The PDMP is under the aegis of a specified statewide regulatory, administrative, or law-enforcement agency. This agency distributes data to individuals who are authorized under state law to receive the information for use in practicing their professions.

System Evolution

1989   Nine established PDMPs began to collect data on Schedule II prescriptions (CII) only, and all used multi-page state-serialized prescription forms. The original form was kept at the pharmacy and the copy was sent to the PDMP for key-punch data entry.

1990s   The Alliance of States with Prescription Monitoring Programs was established with support from the Drug Enforcement Administration (DEA). With its support, PDMPs expanded data collection beyond CIIs, moving toward electronic data capture aided by the American Society for Automation in Pharmacy (ASAP)-published guidelines for standardizing formats for data collection.

2000s   The Harold Rogers Prescription Drug Monitoring Grant Program was created in the U.S. De-

Prescription drug abuse has achieved epidemic proportions in the U.S. during the past decade. The abuses, overdose deaths, and diversion of controlled substance prescription medication are a major public health and safety concern. The PDMD initiative is to encourage **safer prescribing of controlled substances** and to reduce drug abuse and diversion.

partment of Justice, Bureau of Justice Assistance (BJA). The BJA also designated the National Association for Model State Drug Laws (NAMSDL) to assist states in developing PDMP legislation. Later, Congress passed the National All Schedules Prescription Electronic Reporting (NASPER) Act, authorizing additional federal funding for PDMPs.

2012   Forty-nine states had by this year passed legislation to create PDMPs, with operating programs in forty-one. Funding is being made available to enable states to integrate their PDMPs into electronic health records (EHRs) and other health information technology systems to broaden use of PDMP data.

Structure & Terminology

PDMPs enhance the capacity of regulatory and law-enforcement agencies as well as public health officials to collect and analyze controlled-substance prescription data through a centralized database administered by an authorized state agency. The Drug Enforcement Administration (DEA) is not involved with the administration of any state PDMP; however, federal government support for the databases is provided through state grants. The PDMPs are a tool used by the states to: support access to legitimate medical use of controlled substances; identify and deter or prevent drug abuse and diversion; facilitate and encourage the identification, intervention with, and treatment of persons addicted to prescription drugs; and inform public health initiatives through outlining of use and abuse trends.

Most recently, the PDMP-Electronic Health Record (EHR) Integration and Interoperability Expansion grant program aims to help reduce prescription drug misuse and abuse through enhanced utilization of PDMP data without disrupting the healthcare provider's regular workflow. To accomplish this, funding is being made available to integrate PDMP data into existing systems like EHRs and pharmacy dispensing systems with appropriate privacy protections.

Society for Thoracic Surgeons General Thoracic Surgery Database (STS GTSD)

The Society for Thoracic Surgeons (STS)'s General Thoracic Surgery Database (GTSD) is a voluntary initiative to accumulate patient data from cardiothoracic surgical practices nationwide to support quality improvement and patient safety initiatives. All participants sign a contract that requires complete reporting of all cases, and prohibits selective reporting. Although participation in the STS database is voluntary, it is the most widely recognized database to fulfill regulators' and third-party payers' requirements for credentialing and reimbursement for cardiothoracic surgery. Random on-site audits by an independent auditing firm verify accurate data collection; Duke Clinical Research Institute (DCRI) is the data warehouse and analysis center for the Database. Until 2011, outcomes were not publicly released; rather, data were used internally to study, evaluate, and improve cardiothoracic surgery.

System Evolution

1986	The release of raw mortality data for coronary artery bypass grafting (CABG) by the Health Care Financing Agency (HCFA) fueled an effort for a tool suitable for comparison of outcomes.
1987	The STS Standards and Ethics Committee proposed the creation of a comprehensive regis-

In 2011, the STS launched Public Reporting Online, enabling participants to report, if they wished, their **heart bypass surgery** performance.

try. Two years later, an Ad Hoc Committee established a national database for thoracic surgery.

1990   Summit Medical Systems was engaged to develop software for data storage and risk stratification models. In June, the STS National Database was established; by September, it had 50 participants.

1991   Dr. Richard E. Clark, the pioneer who directed the development of the database, published the first report announcing the successful commencement of this endeavor.

1994   The Annals of Thoracic Surgery published the first scientific articles based on material from the database, triggering interest in mining it, and stimulating the formation of the Access and Publications Subcommittee to coordinate use of the data.

1998   Data warehouse functions were transferred from Summit Medical to DCRI to be associated with a reputable academic institution for data analysis and risk stratification.

2011   The Database continued to expand. The STS launched Public Reporting Online, enabling participants to voluntarily report to the public their heart bypass surgery performance. An initiative began to encourage Database participation worldwide by including international participants in the Adult Cardiac Surgery Database.

Structure & Terminology

The STS National Database has three components, each focusing on a different area of cardiothoracic surgery: Adult Cardiac, General Thoracic, and Congenital Heart Surgery. The STS National Database and its quality-assessment activities, development of nationally recognized quality measures, and quality improvement initiatives are all built on, and spring from, more than 5 million surgical records. These records allow the building of identical minimum datasets from patients; outcomes reported are measured systematically using identical definitions across all sites. Some examples of outcomes: risk-adjusted deep sternal wound infection rate, risk-adjusted operative mortality for CABG, anti-platelet medication at discharge.

Besides providing benchmarks for providers, the database is a powerful source that permits the cardiovascular profession to monitor important safety information, detect infrequent complications, and build a clinical research infrastructure crucial to advancing the science surrounding these surgical procedures.

Uniform Ambulatory Care Data Set (UACDS)

The Uniform Ambulatory Care Data Set (UACDS) is a standard dataset for outpatient settings, such as a physician's office, stand-alone health facility, emergency room, or same-day surgery center, or the patient's home. The UACDS was established by the U.S. federal government, through the work of the National Committee on Vital and Health Statistics (NCVHS), with the goal of improving data comparison for ambulatory care settings and a focus on the reason for the healthcare encounter.

System Evolution

1970s   Development of a uniform minimum data set for ambulatory care began in 1972 and was first approved by NCVHS, an external advisory committee to the U.S. Department of Health and Human Services (HHS), in 1975.

1989   A revision by the NCVHS and an Interagency Task Force was widely circulated, but was never officially promulgated by the Department, and remains a recommendation rather than a requirement.

1996   NCVHS completed a report and recommendations on standardizing 42 core health-data elements for enrollment and encounter, and submitted them to the HHS Data Council. This material continues under review within HHS.

Structure & Terminology

The uniform bill, CMS-1500, is the major vehicle for collecting the raw data for the UACDS, which is designed for improvement of ambulatory patient care. The three informational components of the dataset are:

» information that identifies and characterizes the patient;

» information that identifies and characterizes the provider;

» information that identifies and characterizes each encounter between patient and provider.

While the dataset has some of the same elements as the Uniform Hospital Discharge Data Set (UHDDS), such as personal identifier, residence, date of birth, gender, and racial|ethnic background, elements specific to an ambulatory care encounter make this dataset unique. Some examples of these category-specific elements include reason for encounter, problem diagnosis or assessment, place of encounter, and living arrangements.

The UACDS dataset was originally developed to aid in professional review, planning, clarifying curricula objectives, and health services research; however, the benefits of comprehensive and accurate data capture have impact far beyond support of these goals. As an example, the Institute of Medicine (IOM), an independent, nonprofit organization that works outside of government to provide unbiased and authoritative advice to decision-makers and the public, has documented evidence that race and ethnicity are predictors of the quality of care as a result of accurate data capture. The study, "Unequal Treatment: Confronting Racial and Ethnic Disparities in Health Care" (2002) under-scores significant variation in the rates of medical proce-dures by race, even when insurance status, income, age, and severity of conditions are comparable; prompting the IOM's recommendation for reducing racial and ethnic dis-parities in health care including an increased awareness about disparities among the general public, healthcare providers, insurance companies, and policy-makers.

111

This UACDS captures information about care delivered in **numerous outpatient settings** and can provide insights, which can help improve patient care by addressing disparities in providing it.

Uniform Hospital Discharge Data Set (UHDDS)

The Uniform Hospital Discharge Data Set (UHDDS) is the core dataset for hospital reporting. It is the oldest uniform data set used in the United States, and is considered the de facto standard by federal agencies, states, and much of the private sector collecting data on hospital discharges. The standard Uniform Bill (UB) for institutional healthcare providers, known as UB-04, is the major vehicle for collecting the data. The National Committee on Vital and Health Statistics (NCVHS) advises the Department of Health and Human Services (HHS) on the data elements and their definitions, which can be found in the July 31, 1985, Federal Register (Vol. 50, No. 147).

System Evolution

1969   The first U.S. attempt at data uniformity outside vital statistics began with an historic conference at Airlie House in Virginia. The meeting generated a request that the NCVHS develop a uniform minimum data set for hospital discharges; an NCVHS subcommittee was appointed for this project the next year.

1973   The first Uniform Hospital Abstract Minimum Data Set was published after extensive field test and study. While not established as part of Departmental policy until 1980, it was endorsed by several key national organizations in the private sector. The next year, the Department of Health, Education and Welfare initiated the UHDDS to improve the uniformity of hospital discharge data for patients enrolled in Medicaid and Medicare.

1980-90's   Systematic revision continued for several years. NCVHS recommended a revision of the promulgated 1984 UHDDS to Health and Human Services (HHS) in 1992. Recommendations for 42 standardized core health data elements are still under review by HHS.

1991   NCVHS recommended that external cause-of-injury codes (E-codes) become an element of the UHDDS, after becoming convinced of their merits for prevention efforts, and successfully lobbied for the National Uniform Billing Committee to add space on the UB for this purpose.

Structure & Terminology

The official dataset consists of personal identification, date of birth, sex, race and ethnicity, residence, healthcare facility identification number, admission date and type of admission, discharge date, attending physician identification, surgeon identification, principal diagnosis, other diagnoses, principal procedure and dates, other procedures and dates, disposition of patient at discharge, expected payer for most of the bill, and total charge. The UHDDS has elements used in the calculation of the inpatient payment system, so proper application of the guidelines, including sequencing of diagnosis and procedures, is important.

The UHDDS is a prime example of satisfying multiple purposes with a single dataset. A study funded by the Agency for Healthcare Research and Quality (AHRQ) found that the dataset was being used for injury|disease surveillance, public reporting of data for quality improvement and informed purchasing, public health planning, legislation and policy development, and other commercial applications.

The UHDDS is the core dataset for hospital reporting. It is the oldest uniform data set used in the United States, and is considered the *de facto standard* by federal agencies, states, and much of the private sector collecting data on hospital discharges.

United Network for Organ Sharing (UNOS)

The United Network for Organ Sharing (UNOS) is the private, non-profit, scientific and educational organization that manages the USA's organ transplant system. The transplant community is united by the nationwide Organ Procurement and Transplantation Network (OPTN). UNOS, based in Richmond, Virginia, administers the OPTN under contract with the Health Resources and Services Administration (HRSA) of the U.S. Department of Health and Human Services (HHS). UNOS developed an online database system, UNetSM, for the collection, storage, analysis, and publication of all OPTN data pertaining to the patient waiting list, organ matching, and transplants.

System Evolution

1968-1977   UNOS was created as an initiative of the South-Eastern Organ Procurement Foundation (SEOPF). SEOPF implemented the first computer-based organ matching system, the United Network for Organ Sharing.

1984   UNOS was incorporated as an independent, non-profit organization, and separated from the SEOPF. In the same year, the U.S. Congress enacted the National Organ Transplant Act (NOTA), mandating the establishment of the OPTN and of the Scientific Registry of Transplant Recipients (SRTR).

1986   UNOS was awarded the initial OPTN contract on 30 September.

1992   UNOS issued its first comprehensive report on transplant survival rates for all active U.S. transplant centers.

1999   UNet, a secure, internet-based transplant information database system for all organ-matching and management of transplant data, was launched.

2000   HHS published the Final Rule (a federal regulation) for the structure and opera-
        tions of the OPTN.

2006   UNOS launched DonorNetSM, an integrated part of UNet, to increase the effi-
        ciency and accuracy of the organ placement process, replacing faxes and phone
        calls with electronic offers of newly donated organs to transplant hospitals with
        compatible candidates.

Structure & Terminology

All data in the OPTN database is collected via the online web application UNet. Transplant
professionals from hospitals, histocompatibility (tissue-typing) laboratories, and organ-pro-
curement organizations across the country use the application to manage their list of waiting
transplant candidates, access and complete electronic data collection forms, add donor information and run donor-recipient matching lists, and access various transplant data reports
and policies. The data collection forms comprise the largest percentage of the data collected
in the system: 26 different form types contain in the aggregate more than 3,500 data fields.
The system holds data on every organ donation and trans-
plant event that has occurred in the U.S. since October 1,
1987. The SRTR uses this data for its critical role in policy
development through ongoing data analyses designed to
provide the OPTN with information crucial for informed decision-making and policy-setting.

The UNOS system holds data
on every **organ donation
and transplant** event that
has occurred in the U.S.
since October 1, 1987.

Example: OPTN & SRTR Annual Data Report 2011

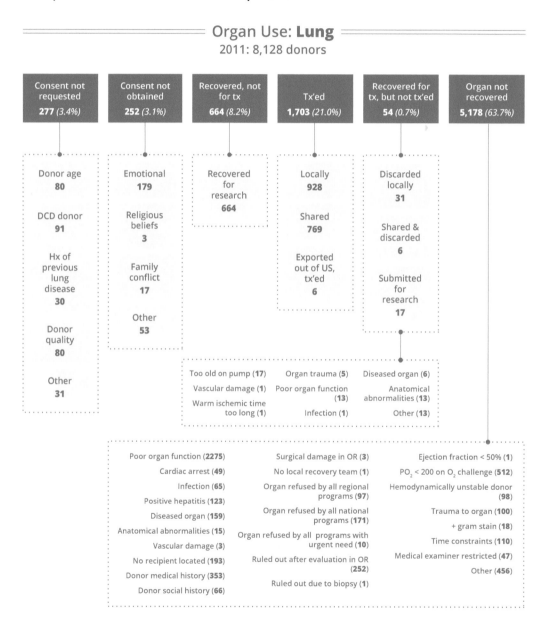

Organ Use: **Lung**
2011: 8,128 donors

Consent not requested	Consent not obtained	Recovered, not for tx	Tx'ed	Recovered for tx, but not tx'ed	Organ not recovered
277 *(3.4%)*	**252** *(3.1%)*	**664** *(8.2%)*	**1,703** *(21.0%)*	**54** *(0.7%)*	**5,178** *(63.7%)*

Consent not requested
Donor age
80

DCD donor
91

Hx of previous lung disease
30

Donor quality
80

Other
31

Consent not obtained
Emotional
179

Religious beliefs
3

Family conflict
17

Other
53

Recovered, not for tx
Recovered for research
664

Tx'ed
Locally
928

Shared
769

Exported out of US, tx'ed
6

Recovered for tx, but not tx'ed
Discarded locally
31

Shared & discarded
6

Submitted for research
17

Too old on pump (**17**)   Organ trauma (**5**)   Diseased organ (**6**)
Vascular damage (**1**)   Poor organ function (**13**)   Anatomical abnormalities (**13**)
Warm ischemic time too long (**1**)   Infection (**1**)   Other (**13**)

Poor organ function (**2275**)   Surgical damage in OR (**3**)   Ejection fraction < 50% (**1**)
Cardiac arrest (**49**)   No local recovery team (**1**) PO_2 < 200 on O_2 challenge (**512**)
Infection (**65**)   Organ refused by all regional programs (**97**)   Hemodynamically unstable donor (**98**)
Positive hepatitis (**123**)   Organ refused by all national programs (**171**)   Trauma to organ (**100**)
Diseased organ (**159**)   Organ refused by all programs with urgent need (**10**)   + gram stain (**18**)
Anatomical abnormalities (**15**)   Ruled out after evaluation in OR (**252**)   Time constraints (**110**)
Vascular damage (**3**)   Ruled out due to biopsy (**1**)   Medical examiner restricted (**47**)
No recipient located (**193**)   Other (**456**)
Donor medical history (**353**)
Donor social history (**66**)

United States Health Information Knowledgebase (USHIK) and Meaningful Use (MU)

The United States Health Information Knowledgebase (USHIK) is an online, publicly accessible registry and repository of healthcare-related data, metadata, and standards, including Meaningful Use (MU). MU is a collection of measurable benchmarks that providers must meet to qualify for Electronic Health Record (EHR) incentive payments, proving that they are "meaningfully using" their EHR's by achieving thresholds for a number of objectives. USHIK is funded and directed by the Agency for Healthcare Research and Quality (AHRQ), with management support in partnership with the Centers for Medicare & Medicaid Services (CMS).

System Evolution

2009   The American Recovery and Reinvestment Act (ARRA) law allocated $19.2 billion to increase the use of EHR's by physicians and hospitals; this mandate was included in a portion of the bill called the Health Information Technology for Economic and Clinical Health Act (HITECH). Meaningful Use is a core requirement of HITECH, serving its larger goal of the migration of health reform toward value-based healthcare through increased access to clinical infor-

The United States Health Information Knowledgebase (USHIK) is an online, publicly accessible registry and repository of healthcare-related data, metadata, and standards, including **Meaningful Use** (MU).

mation for all stakeholders, thereby improving quality, patient outcomes and cost containment. MU incentive programs are to evolve in three steps with increasing requirements for participation.

2011-2012 Stage 1 focused on providers capturing structured patient data in the EHR and electronically sharing that data either with the patient or with other healthcare professionals.

2014 Stage 2 is projected to advance clinical processes including quality measures and their value sets; there are also high expectations for health-information exchange.

2016 Stage 3 foresees improved outcomes and greater interoperability.

Structure & Terminology

USHIK's Meaningful Use portal acts as a consolidated resource for finding information on the Meaningful Use Core and Menu Measures as well as retrieving data on Clinical Quality Measures (CQM) and Value Sets. Succinctly, Core and Menu Measures are objectives, like E-prescribing or Computerized Provider Order Entry (CPOE) capabilities, that providers must prove substantive use of. CQM's have been defined as measures of processes, experience, and|or outcomes of patient care, observations or treatment that relate to one or more of the Institute of Medicine (IOM) domains of health care quality (as expressed by modifiers such as "effective," "safe," "efficient," "patient-centered," "equitable," "timely"). Examples of CQM are adult weight screening, cervical cancer screening, and or childhood immunization status. Value Sets provide lists of numerical values and individual names from standard vocabularies that define clinical concepts—for example, diabetes. Below are listed definitions of "Meaningful Use" of Core and Menu Measures. "EP" is eligible profession; "HP," hospital:

Stage 1 EP: 15 (Core Measures) + 5 out of 10 (Menu Measures) + 6 (CQMs) = Meaningful Use

Stage 1 HP: 14 (Core Measures) + 5 out of 10 (Menu Measures) + 6 (CQMs) = Meaningful Use

Stage 2 EP: 17 (Core Measures) + 3 out of 5 (Menu Measures) + 12 (CQMs) = Meaningful Use

Stage 2 HP: 16 (Core Measures) + 2 out of 4 (Menu Measures) + 24 (CQMs) = Meaningful Use

Besides Meaningful Use Measures Metadata (MUMM), other initiatives (portals) supported by USHIK include: Standards Developing Organizations (SDO), Patient Safety Common Formats–Center for Quality Improvement and Patient Safety (CQuIPS), Health Information Technology Standards Panel (HITSP), All-Payer Claims Databases (APCD), and Standards and Interoperability Framework (S&I).

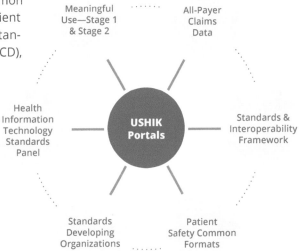

Six USHIK Information Models for Selected Data Elements in USHIK

Appendix

A (Virtually Interminable) List of Useful Acronyms

ACS . . . . American College of Surgeons

AHA . . . . American Hospital Association

AHCPR . . . . . . Agency for Health Care Policy and Research

AHRQ . . . . . . Agency for Healthcare Research and Quality

AJCC . . . . American Joint Committee for Cancer

ALS . . . . Amyotrophic Lateral Sclerosis

ALSFRS-R . . . . ALS Functional Rating Scale-Revised (see ALS)

AMA . . . . American Medical Association

AMI . . . . Acute Myocardial Infarction

AMLOS . . . . . . Arithmetic Mean Length of Stay

AMSI . . . . APACHE Medical Systems, Inc.

ANA . . . . American Nurses Association

AORN . . . . . . Association of periOperative Registered Nurses

APA . . . . American Psychiatric Association

APACHE . . . . . Acute Physiology and Chronic Health Evaluation

APCD . . . . All-Payer Claims Databases

APS . . . . Acute Physiology Score

ARRA . . . . American Recovery and Reinvestment Act

ASA . . . . American Society of Anesthesiologists

ASAP . . . . American Society for Automation in Pharmacy

ASMBS . . . . . . American Society for Metabolic and Bariatric Surgery

BBA . . . . Balanced Budget Act

BJA . . . . Bureau of Justice Assistance

BOLD . . . . . . Bariatric Outcomes Longitudinal Database
BSCOE . . . . . . Bariatric Surgery Centers of Excellence
CABG . . . . . . Coronary Artery Bypass Grafting
caBIG . . . . . . Cancer Biomedical Informatics Grid
CAHPS . . . . . . Consumer Assessment of Healthcare Providers and Systems
CARE . . . . Continuity Assessment Record Evaluation
CBTRUS . . . . . Central Brain Tumor Registry of the United States
CCC . . . . Clinical Care Classification (System)
CECS . . . . Center for the Evaluative Clinical Sciences
CF . . . . Conversion Factor
CHIP . . . . Children's Health Insurance Program
CHIPRA . . . . . Children's Health Insurance Program Reauthorization Act
CIS . . . . Carcinoma in situ
CMS . . . . Centers for Medicare and Medicaid Services
COE . . . . Center of Excellence
CPOE . . . . . . Computerized Provider Order Entry
CPR . . . . Customary, Prevailing and Reasonable
CPT . . . . Current Procedural Terminology
CQM . . . . Clinical Quality Measures
CQuIPS . . . . . Center for Quality Improvement and Patient Safety
CUI . . . . Concept Unique Identifiers
DAP . . . . Dartmouth Atlas Project
DCRI . . . . Duke Clinical Research Institute
DEA . . . . Drug Enforcement Administration
DEEDS . . . . . . Data Elements for Emergency Department Systems
DME . . . . Durable Medical Equipment
DMEPOS . . . . . Durable Medical Equipment, Prosthetics, Orthotics and Supplies
DRC . . . . Data Resource Center for Child and Adolescent Health
DRG . . . . Diagnonsis Related Groups
DRLS . . . . Drug Registration and Listing System
DSM . . . . Diagnosis Statistical Manual

DUA . . . . Data Use Agreement

E&M . . . . Evaluation and Management (Codes)

ECRI . . . . Emergency Care Research Institute

ED . . . . Emergency Department

EHR . . . . Electronic Health Record

FDA . . . . Food and Drug Administration

FDCA . . . . Food, Drug and Cosmetic Act

FIGO . . . . International Federation of Gynecology and Obstetrics (originally a Swiss acronym)

GAF . . . . Global Assessment of Functioning

GIS . . . . Geographical Information System

GMLOS . . . . . Geometric Mean Length of Stay

GPCI . . . . Geographic Practice Cost Index

GTSD . . . . General Thoracic Surgery Database

HAVEN . . . . . . Home Assessment and Validation and Entry

HCAHPS . . . . . Hospital Consumer Assessment of Healthcare Providers and Systems

HCFA . . . . Health Care Financing Administration (Now CMS)

HCPCS . . . . . . Healthcare Common Procedure Coding System

HCUP . . . . . . Healthcare Cost and Utilization Project

HEDIS . . . . . . Healthcare Effectiveness Data and Information Set

HHRG . . . . . . Home Health Resource Group

HHS . . . . Health and Human Services

HIPAA . . . . . . Health Insurance Portability and Accountability Act

HITECH . . . . . Health Information Technology for Economic and Clinical Health (Act)

HITSP . . . . . . Health Information Technology Standards Panel

HL7 . . . . Health Level Seven

HLGT . . . . High-Level Group Term

HLT . . . . High-Level Term

HMO . . . . Health Maintenance Organization

HRSA . . . . Health Resources and Services Administration

ICD . . . . International Classification of Disease

ICH . . . . International Conference on Harmonization
ICN . . . . International Council of Nurses
ICNP . . . . International Classification for Nursing Practice
ICU . . . . Intensive Care Unit
IFPMA . . . . . . International Federation of Pharmaceutical Manufacturers and Associations
IHTSDO . . . . . International Heath Terminology Standards Development Organization
IOM . . . . Institute of Medicine
IPPS . . . . Inpatient Prospective Payment System
IQR . . . . Inpatient Quality Reporting
IVR . . . . Interactive Voice Recognition
JC . . . . Joint Commission
JCAHO . . . . . . Joint Commission on Accreditation of Healthcare Organizations
KID . . . . Kids' In-patient Database
LDS . . . . Limited Data Set
LLT . . . . Lowest-Level Terms
LOINC . . . . . . Logical Observation Identifiers Names and Codes
LOS . . . . Length of Stay
MAC . . . . Medicare Administrative Contractors
MBSAQIP . . . . Metabolic and Bariatric Surgery Accreditation and Quality Improvement Program
MCA . . . . Medicines Control Agency
MDC . . . . Major Diagnostic Category
MDS . . . . Minimum Data Set
MEDPAR . . . . . Medicare Provider Analysis and Review
MEDDRA . . . . . Medical Dictionary for Regulatory Activities
MeSH . . . . . . Medical Subject Headings
MQA . . . . Medicare Quality Assurance
MRI . . . . Midwest Research Institute
MS-DRG . . . . . Medicare Severity-Diagnosis Related Groups
MSIS . . . . Medicaid Statistical Information System
MSSO . . . . . . Maintenance and Support Services Organization

MTOS . . . . . . Major Trauma Outcome Study
MU . . . . Meaningful Use
MUMM . . . . . Meaningful Use Measures Metadata
NAMSDL . . . . . National Association for Model State Drug Laws
NANDA . . . . . North American Nursing Diagnoses Association
NAPHSIS . . . . . National Association of Public Health Statistics and Information Systems
NASPER . . . . . National All Schedules Prescription Electronic Reporting
NCH . . . . National Claims History
NCHS . . . . . . National Center for Health Statistics
NCI . . . . National Cancer Institute
NCIP . . . . National Cancer Informatics Program
NCIPC . . . . . . National Center for Injury Prevention and Control
NCNQI . . . . . . National Database of Nursing Quality Indicators
NCQA . . . . . . National Committee for Quality Assurance
NCRA . . . . . . National Cancer Registrars Association
NCVHS . . . . . . National Committee on Vital and Health Statistics
NDC . . . . National Drug Codes
NDF-RT . . . . . National Drug File-Reference Terminology
NDI . . . . National Death Index
NDNQI . . . . . . National Database of Nursing Quality Indicators
NEDS . . . . Nationwide Emergency Department Sample
NHAMCS . . . . National Hospital Ambulatory Medical Care Survey
NHCS . . . . . . National Hospital Care Survey
NHDS . . . . . . National Hospital Discharge Survey
NHQR . . . . . . National Healthcare Quality Report
NIC . . . . Nursing Interventions Classification
NIH . . . . National Institutes of Health
NIS . . . . Nationwide Inpatient Sample
NLM . . . . National Library of Medicine
NLP . . . . Natural Language Processing
NOC . . . . Nursing Outcomes Classification

NOTA . . . . . . National Organ Transplant Act

NPCR. . . . . . . National Program of Cancer Registries

NQF . . . . National Quality Forum

NSCH . . . . . . National Survey of Children's Health

NS-CSHCN. . . . National Survey of Children with Special Health Care Needs

NSP . . . . National Sample Program

NSQIP . . . . . . National Surgical Quality Improvement Program

NTDB . . . . . . National Trauma Data Bank

NTDS. . . . . . . National Trauma Data Standard

NTR . . . . National Trauma Registry

NVSS . . . . National Vital Statistics System

OASIS . . . . . . Outcome and Assessment Information Set

OBRA . . . . . . Omnibus Budget Reconciliation Act

OPTN . . . . . . Organ Procurement and Transplantation Network

PDMP . . . . . . Prescription Drug Monitoring Program

PLM . . . . PatientsLikeMe

PNDS . . . . . . Perioperative Nursing Data Set

PPACA . . . . . . Patient Protection and Affordable Care Act

PPRC. . . . . . . Physician Payment Review Comission

PPS. . . . . Prospective Payment System

PQMP . . . . . . Pediatric Quality Measures Program

PRO . . . . Peer Review Organization

PUF . . . . Public Use Files

QI . . . . Quality Indicator

QIES . . . . Quality Improvement Evaluation System

QIO. . . . . Quality Improvement Organization

RAI . . . . Resident Assessment Instrument

RAP . . . . Resident Assessment Protocol

RBRVS . . . . . . Resource-Based Relative Value Scale

RELMA . . . . . . Regenstrief LOINC Mapping Assistant (See LOINC)

ResDAC . . . . . Research Data Assistance Center

RHQDAPU . . . . Reporting Hospital Quality Data for Annual Payment Update
RIF . . . . Research Identifiable Files
RUC . . . . RVS Update Committee (See RBRVS)
RUG . . . . Resource Utilization Group
RVU . . . . Relative Value Units
RXAUI . . . . . . RxNorm Atom Unique Identifier
RXCUI . . . . . . RxNorm Concept Unique Identifier
S&I . . . . Standards and Interoperability (Framework)
SASD . . . . State Ambulatory Surgery Databases
SCIP . . . . Surgical Care Improvement Project
SCR . . . . Surgical Clinical Reviewer
SDO . . . . Standards Developing Organizations
SEDD . . . . State Emergency Department Databases
SEER . . . . Surveillance, Epidemiology and End Results
SEOPF . . . . . . South-Eastern Organ Procurement Foundation
SID . . . . State Inpatient Databases
SMQ . . . . Standardized MedDRA Queries (See MEDDRA)
SNF . . . . Skilled Nursing Facilities
SNL . . . . Standardized Nursing Languages
SNOMED . . . . Systematized Nomenclature of Medicine
SNOMED-CT . . Systematized Nomenclature of Medicine—Clinical Terms
SNOMED-RT . . . Systematized Nomenclature of Medicine—Reference Terminology
SNOP . . . . . . Systematized Nomenclature of Pathology
SOC . . . . System Organ Class
SRTR . . . . Scientific Registry of Transplant Recipients
STS . . . . Society for Thoracic Surgeons
STS GTSD . . . . Society for Thoracic Surgeons General Thoracic Surgery Database
TDI . . . . The Dartmouth Institute
TNM . . . . Tumor, Node, Metastasis
TOC . . . . Type of Code
UACDS . . . . . . Uniform Ambulatory Care Data Set

UB . . . . Universal Bill
UHDDS . . . . . Uniform Hospital Discharge Data Set
UICC . . . . International Union Against Cancer (originally a French acronym)
UMDNS . . . . . Universal Medical Device Nomenclature System
UMLS . . . . . . Unified Medical Language System
UMLSKS . . . . . UMLS Knowledge Source Server (see UMLS)
UNOS . . . . . . United Network for Organ Sharing
UPDRS . . . . . . Unified Parkinson's Disease Rating Scale
USHIK . . . . . . United States Health Information Knowledgebase
VA . . . . Veterans Administration
VBP . . . . Value-Based Purchasing
WHO . . . . World Health Organizaton

Annotated Bibliography

Below is a list of the sources used to write this book. These sources should be read and referred to in light of the following observations.

Without question, real healthcare reform and improvement will be driven by data that correctly captures the information required to improve the structures, processes, and outcomes of care. However, defining and capturing the right data in the right way—and creating consensus on what that is across multiple stakeholders with numerous (often conflicting) viewpoints can be most politely defined as "herding cats." One result of these different points of view and interpretations is a proliferation of rapidly evolving data and databases, often focused on a particular group or constituent's area of knowledge, skills, or interest.

Further, the rate of creation, adoption, and use of these data and databases has outpaced— rendering obsolete and often permanently replacing—many printed textbooks that traditionally would be used as reference sources. A wide variety of websites have provided valuable current context for this book; but as many readers know, these sites are not always closely and reliably vetted, revised, or updated by experts in the field, and the sites appear, change coordinates, and|or vanish with daunting speed and frequency. Organizations, institutions, publications, government entities and agencies, reference works, and individual experts, practitioners, and scholars provided a great deal of valuable and substantive information while this book was being written, and every attempt was made to verify the solidity and legitimacy of each source. On other occasions, it was not possible to evaluate, give credit for, or sometimes even find original sources.

If you discover that we have overlooked or misstated an important facet of healthcare classification systems or databases, please let us know. Future editions of the book will improve thanks to your input.

Acute Physiology and Chronic Health Evaluation (APACHE)

» Burton GG. APACHE II vs APACHE III Scoring. Medscape Critical Care [Internet]. 2001 May 22 [cited 2012 March 26]; Available from: http://www.medscape.com/viewarticle/412361

» Knaus WA. APACHE 1978-2001: the development of a quality assurance system based on prognosis: milestones and personal reflections. Arch Surg. 2002 Jan;137(1):37–41.

» Knaus WA, Draper EA, Wagner D, Zimmerman J. APACHE II: A severity of disease classification system : Critical Care Medicine. Critical Care Medicine [Internet]. 1985 Oct [cited 2012 March 25];13(10). Available from: http://journals.lww.com/ccmjournal/Fulltext/1985/10000/APACHE_II__A_severity_of_disease_classification.9.aspx

» Manganaro L, Stark M, editors. APACHE Foundations User Guide. Cerner Corporation; 2010.

American Society of Anesthesiologists (ASA) Physical Status Classification System

» ASA Physical Status Classification System [Internet]. [cited 2012 Nov 26]. Available from: http://www.asahq.org/Home/For-Members/Clinical-Information/ASA-Physical-Status-Classification-System

» Daabiss M. American Society of Anaesthesiologists physical status classification. Indian J Anaesth [Internet]. 2011 [cited 2012 Nov 21];55(2):111–5. Available from: http://www.ncbi.nlm.nih.gov/pmc/articles/PMC3106380/

» Wolters U, Wolf T, Stützer H, Schröder T. ASA classification and perioperative variables as predictors of postoperative outcome. Br J Anaesth. 1996 Aug;77(2):217–22.

Apgar Score (APGAR)

» APGAR V. A proposal for a new method of evaluation of the newborn infant. Curr Res Anesth Analg. 1953 Aug;32(4):260–7.

» Butterfield J. Practical Epigram of Apgar Score. Pediatrics [Internet]. 1989 Nov 1 [cited 2012 Mar 25];84(5):778–778. Available from: http://pediatrics.aappublications.org/content/84/5/778

» Dastur AE, Tank PD. Virginia Apgar and Evaluation of the Newborn Infant. J Obstet Gynecol India. 2008 Aug;58(4).

» Pediatrics AA of, Newborn C on F and, Gynecologists AC of O and, Practice C on O. The Apgar Score. Pediatrics [Internet]. 2006 Apr 1 [cited 2012 Mar 26];117(4):1444–7. Available from: http://pediatrics.aappublications.org/content/117/4/1444

» Sideras J. APGAR scoring for newborn delivery [Internet]. EMS1. [cited 2012 Mar 21]. Available from: http://www.ems1.com/ems-news/849911-APGAR-scoring-for-newborn-delivery/

Bariatric Outcomes Longitudinal Database (BOLD)

» Bariatric & Metabolic Surgery | Surgical Review Corporation [Internet]. Surgical Review Corporation. [cited 2012 Jun 18]. Available from: http://www.surgicalreview.org/bold/bariatric/

» Blackstone R. Collecting and Using Data: Beyond the First Data Registry

» ASMBS News and Update: April 2012 [Internet]. Bariatric Times. [cited 2012 Apr 29]. Available from: http://bariatrictimes.com/2012/04/16/april-asmbs-news-and-update/

» Blackstone R. Metabolic Surgery for Type 2 Diabetes | American Society for Metabolic and Bariatric Surgery [Internet]. 2012 [cited 2013 Feb 14]. Available from: http://asmbs.org/2012/04/metabolic-surgery-for-type-2-diabetes/

» Blackstone R. Part 2: The American Society for Metabolic and Bariatric Surgery Bariatric Surgery Quality Improvement Program (ASMBS NBSQIP)--On what outcome measure should the ASMBS base accreditation? [Internet]. American Society for Metabolic and Bariatric Surgery; 2012. Available from: http://s3.amazonaws.com/publicASMBS/Items_of_Interest/Segment%202.2.pdf

» DeMaria EJ, Pate V, Warthen M, Winegar DA. Baseline data from American Society for Metabolic and Bariatric Surgery-designated Bariatric Surgery Centers of Excellence using the Bariatric Outcomes Longitudinal Database. Surg Obes Relat Dis. 2010 Aug;6(4):347–55.

» Iezzoni LI, editor. Risk Adjustment for Measuring Healthcare Outcomes, Third Edition. 3rd ed. Health Administration Press; 2003.

Cancer Registry

» CDC - Cancer - National Program of Cancer Registries (NPCR) [Internet]. [cited 2012 Jul 10]. Available from: http://www.cdc.gov/cancer/npcr/

» Lowenstein C. Cancer Registries and Medical Records: Rich Data Resources [Internet]. 2010 [cited 2012 Jul 16]. Available from: http://www.umb.edu/editor_uploads/ images/U54%20Seminar-Ca%20Registries%20and%20MR%20Review%2010-12-11. ppt

» NCIP - NCI BioMedical Informatics Blog [Internet]. National Cancer Informatics Program. [cited 2013 Mar 23]. Available from: http://ncip.nci.nih.gov/blog/tag/ncip-2/

» NCRA - National Cancer Registrars Association [Internet]. National Cancer Registrars Association. [cited 2012 Jul 12]. Available from: http://www.ncra-usa.org/i4a/ pages/index.cfm?pageid=3277

» Ovarian Cancer Registry [Internet]. The Gilda Radner Familial. [cited 2012 Jul 10]. Available from: http://ovariancancer.com/

» SEER Web Site [Internet]. National Cancer Institute. [cited 2012 Jul 10]. Available from: http://www.seer.cancer.gov/

Centers for Medicare & Medicaid Services (CMS) Core Measures

» Chassin MR, Loeb JM, Schmaltz SP, Wachter RM. Accountability Measures — Using Measurement to Promote Quality Improvement. New England Journal of Medicine [Internet]. 2010 [cited 2013 Feb 26];363(7):683–8. Available from: http://www.nejm. org/doi/full/10.1056/NEJMsb1002320

» CMS Makes Changes to Improve Quality of Care During Hospital Inpatient Stays [Internet]. CMS.gov. [cited 2013 May 1]. Available from: http://www.cms.gov/apps/

media/press/factsheet.asp?Counter=4422&intNumPerPage=10&checkDate=&-
checkKey=&srchType=1&numDays=3500&srchOpt=0&srchData=&keyword-
Type=All&chkNewsType=6&intPage=&showAll=&pYear=&year=&desc=&cboOrder=-
date&goback=.gde_954567_member_141950502

» CMS: Roadmap for Implementing Value Driven Healthcare in the Traditional Medi-
care-For-Service Program [Internet]. Centers for Medicare & Medicaid Services;
[cited 2013 May 1]. Available from: http://www.cms.gov/Medicare/Quality-Initia-
tives-Patient-Assessment-Instruments/QualityInitiativesGenInfo/downloads/vb-
proadmap_oea_1-16_508.pdf

» Schmaltz SP, Williams SC, Chassin MR, Loeb JM, Wachter RM. Hospital Performance
Trends on National Quality Measures and the Association With Joint Commission
Accreditation. J Hosp Med [Internet]. 2011 Oct [cited 2013 Feb 26];6(8):454–61.
Available from: http://www.ncbi.nlm.nih.gov/pmc/articles/PMC3265714/

» Specifications Manual for National Hospital Inpatient Quality Measures Version 2.2
[Internet]. Available from: http://www.qualitynet.org/

» Specifications Manual for National Hospital Inpatient Quality Measures Version 2.2
[Internet]. Available from: http://www.qualitynet.org/

» Surgical Care Improvement Project [Internet]. The Joint Commission. 2012
[cited 2103 Mar 26]. Available from: http://www.jointcommission.org/
surgical_care_improvement_project/

Current Procedural Terminology (CPT)

» CPT - Current Procedural Terminology [Internet]. American Medical Association.
[cited 2012 Jan 21]. Available from: http://www.ama-assn.org/ama/pub/physi-
cian-resources/solutions-managing-your-practice/coding-billing-insurance/cpt.page

» Giannangelo K. Healthcare Code Sets, Clinical Terminologies, and Classification
Systems. 2nd ed. AHIMA; 2009.

» Wager KA, Lee FW, Glaser JP. Health Care Information Systems: A Practical Approach for Health Care Management. 2nd ed. Jossey-Bass; 2009.

Dartmouth Atlas Project (DAP)

» Dartmouth Atlas of Health Care [Internet]. [cited 2013 Jan 16]. Available from: http://www.dartmouthatlas.org/

» Skinner J, Fisher E. Reflections on Geographic Variations in US Health Care. 2010 [cited 2013 Feb 1]; Available from: http://www.researchgate.net/publication/228922126_Reflections_on_Geographic_Variations_in_US_Health_Care

» What Is the Dartmouth Atlas of Health Care and Why Is It So Significant? The Medicare Newsgroup [Internet]. [cited 2013 Jan 17]; Available from: http://medicare-newsgroup.com/news/medicare-faqs/individual-faq?faqId=8dd105d2-1cce-4c46-a0be-910f19ba9a17

Data Elements for Emergency Department Systems (DEEDS)

» Data Elements for Emergency Department Systems, Version 1 [Internet]. National Center for Injury Prevention and Control of the Centers for Disease Control and Prevention; 1997 [cited 2012 Oct 13]. Available from: http://www.cdc.gov/ncipc/pub-res/pdf/deeds.pdf

» DEEDS Publication - National Center for Injury Prevention and Control [Internet]. CDC. [cited 2012 Oct 15]. Available from: http://www.cdc.gov/ncipc/pub-res/deedspage.htm

» Pollock DA, Adams DL, Bernardo LM, Bradley V, Brandt MD, Davis TE, et al. Data Elements for Emergency Department Systems, Release 1.0 (DEEDS): A Summary Report. Annals of Emergency Medicine [Internet]. 1998 Feb [cited 2012 Oct 13];31(2):264–73. Available from: http://www.annemergmed.com/article/S0196-0644(98)70317-8/abstract

» Pollock DA. Data Elements for Emergency Department Systems (DEEDS) [Internet]. 1999 [cited 2012 Oct 14]. Available from: http://www.ncvhs.hhs.gov/990517t2.htm

Diagnosis-Related Groups (DRG)

» Hospital Acute Inpatient Services Payment System [Internet]. MedPAC; 2012 [cited 2012 Feb 1]. Available from: http://www.medpac.gov/documents/MedPAC_Payment_Basics_12_hospital.pdf

» Medicare Hospital Prospective Payment System: How DRG Rates Are Calculated and Updated [Internet]. Office of Inspector General Office of Evaluation and Inspections Region IX; 2001 [cited 2012 Feb 9]. Available from: http://oig.hhs.gov/oei/reports/oei-09-00-00200.pdf

» White WD, editor. Compelled by data: John D. Thompson: nurse, health services researcher, and health administration educator. New Haven, Conn.: Dept. of Epidemiology and Public Health, Yale School of Medicine, Yale University]; 2003.

Diagnostic and Statistical Manual of Mental Disorders (DSM)

» Association AP. Diagnostic and Statistical Manual of Mental Disorders, 4th Edition, Text Revision. 4th ed. American Psychiatric Association; 2000.

» DSM: History of the Manual | psychiatry.org [Internet]. American Psychiatric Association. [cited 2013 Mar 22]. Available from: http://www.psychiatry.org/practice/dsm/dsm-history-of-the-manual

» DSM-5 Development [Internet]. American Psychiatric Association. [cited 2013 Mar 22]. Available from: http://www.dsm5.org/Pages/Default.aspx

» Gupta P. Controversial changes to stay in DSM-5. Salon [Internet]. [cited 2012 Apr 10]; Available from: http://www.salon.com/2012/12/02/controversial_changes_to_stay_in_dsm_5/

Geomedicine | Geocoding

» Bowman CA, Bobrowsky PT, Selinus O. Medical geology: new relevance in the earth sciences. 2003 Dec [cited 2012 Apr 22];26(4). Available from: http://www.medicalgeology.org/pages/members/publications/Popular science/Medical Geology.

» Dartmouth Atlas of Health Care [Internet]. [cited 2012 Apr 22]. Available from: http://www.dartmouthatlas.org/

» Davenhall W. Geomedicine [Internet]. TEDMED; 2009 [cited 2012 Apr 23]. Available from: http://www.ted.com/talks/bill_davenhall_your_health_depends_on_where_you_live.html

» Davenhall W. Geomedicine: Geography and Personal Health [Internet]. ERSI; 2012. Available from: http://www.esri.com/industries/health/geomedicine/~/media/Files/Pdfs/library/ebooks/geomedicine.pdf

» Holmes AD, Pigott MG, Packard WH. The Effect of Supplementary Iodine on the Nutritive Value of Chick Rations Four Figures. J. Nutr. [Internet]. 1934 Nov 1 [cited 2012 Apr 22];8(5):583–95. Available from: http://jn.nutrition.org/content/8/5/583

» Hoyt RE, Yoshihashi A. Medical Informatics: Practical Guide for Healthcare and Information Technology Professionals Fourth Edition. 4th ed. lulu.com; 2010.

» Kistemann T, Dangendorf F, Schweikart J. New perspectives on the use of Geographical Information Systems (GIS) in environmental health sciences. Int J Hyg Environ Health. 2002 Apr;205(3):169–81.

» Lag J. Geomedicine. 1st ed. CRC Press; 1990.

» Okerson B. SAS Maps as Tools to Display and Clarify Healthcare Outcome [Internet]. 2010 [cited 2012 Apr 25]. Available from: http://support.sas.com/resources/papers/proceedings10/211-2010.pdf

Healthcare Common Procedure Coding System (HCPCS)

» Giannangelo K. Healthcare Code Sets, Clinical Terminologies, and Classification Systems. 2nd ed. AHIMA; 2009.

» HCPCS - General Information - Centers for Medicare & Medicaid Services [Internet]. CMS.gov. [cited 2012 Jan 23]. Available from: http://www.cms.gov/Medicare/Coding/MedHCPCSGenInfo/index.html?redirect=/medhcpcsgeninfo/

Healthcare Cost and Utilization Project (HCUP)

» Health, United States, 2009 with Special Feature on Medical Technology [Internet]. National Center for Health Statistics; 2009. Available from: http://www.cdc.gov/nchs/data/hus/hus09.pdf

» Healthcare Cost and Utilization Project (HCUP) | Agency for Healthcare Research & Quality (AHRQ) [Internet]. [cited 2013 Jan 31]. Available from: http://www.ahrq.gov/research/data/hcup/index.html

» Healthcare Cost and Utilization Project, State Inpatient Databases (HCUP (SID)) - Health Indicators Warehouse [Internet]. [cited 2013 Jan 31]. Available from: http://healthindicators.gov/Resources/DataSources/HCUP-SID_54/Profile

Healthcare Effectiveness Data and Information Set (HEDIS)

» McPartland G. A History of Total Health. [Internet]. 2012 Mar 21 [cited 2012 Jun 22]; Available from: http://www.kaiserpermanentehistory.org/tag/kaiser-permanente-quality-assurance/

» NCQA: HEDIS Measures [Internet]. [cited 2012 Jun 11]. Available from: http://www.ncqa.org/HEDISQualityMeasurement/HEDISMeasures.aspx

» The State of Health Care Quality: Reform, The Quality Agenda and Resource Use [Internet]. The National Committee for Quality Assurance; 2010. Available from: http://www.ncqa.org/portals/0/state%20of%20health%20care/2010/sohc%202010%20-%20full2.pdf

Hospital Consumer Assessment of Healthcare Providers and Systems (HCAHPS)

» HCAHPS - Hospital Survey [Internet]. [cited 2013 Jan 23]. Available from: http://www.hcahpsonline.org/home.aspx

» Hospital Compare Data Overview [Internet]. [cited 2013 Jan 23]. Available from: http://www.medicare.gov/hospitalcompare/Data/AboutData/About.aspx

» HospitalHCAHPSFactSheet201007.pdf [Internet]. CMS; [cited 2013 Jan 24]. Available from: http://www.cms.gov/Medicare/Quality-Initiatives-Patient-Assessment-Instruments/HospitalQualityInits/downloads/HospitalHCAHPSFactSheet201007.pdf

International Classification of Diseases (ICD)

» History of the development of the ICD [Internet]. World Health Organization; [cited 2012 Mar 3]. Available from: http://www.who.int/classifications/icd/en/HistoryOfICD.pdf

» Hoyt RE, Yoshihashi A. Medical Informatics: Practical Guide for Healthcare and Information Technology Professionals Fourth Edition. 4th ed. lulu.com; 2010.

» Moriyama I, Loy R, Robb-Smith A. History of the statistical classification of diseases and causes of death [Internet]. 2011 [cited 2012 Mar 4]. Available from: http://www.cdc.gov/nchs/data/misc/classification_diseases2011.pdf

Logical Observation Identifiers Names and Codes (LOINC)

» Giannangelo K. Healthcare Code Sets, Clinical Terminologies, and Classification Systems. 2nd ed. AHIMA; 2009.

» Hoyt RE, Yoshihashi A. Medical Informatics: Practical Guide for Healthcare and Information Technology Professionals Fourth Edition. 4th ed. lulu.com; 2010.

» LOINC Background — LOINC [Internet]. [cited 2012 Nov 3]. Available from: http://loinc.org/background

MEDCIN

» Brown SH, Rosenbloom ST, Bauer BA, Wahner-Roedler D, Froehling DA, Bailey KR, et al. Direct Comparison of MEDCIN® and SNOMED CT® for Representation of a General Medical Evaluation Template. AMIA Annu Symp Proc [Internet]. 2007 [cited 2012 Feb 17];2007:75–9. Available from: http://www.ncbi.nlm.nih.gov/pmc/articles/PMC2655894/

» Hoyt RE, Yoshihashi A. Medical Informatics: Practical Guide for Healthcare and Information Technology Professionals Fourth Edition. 4th ed. lulu.com; 2010.

» Peter Goltra: Executive Profile & Biography - Businessweek [Internet]. Businessweek.com. [cited 2012 Feb 20]. Available from: http://investing.businessweek.com/research/stocks/private/person.asp?personId=45788672&privcapId=8186225&previousCapId=8186225&previousTitle=Medicomp%20Systems,%20Inc

» 2012AB MEDCIN Source Information [Internet]. [cited 2012 Feb 20]. Available from: http://www.nlm.nih.gov/research/umls/sourcereleasedocs/current/MEDCIN/

Medical Dictionary for Regulatory Activities (MedDRA)

» Introductory Guide: MedDRA Version 14.0 [Internet]. World Health Organization; 2011 [cited 2012 May 26]. Available from: http://www.who.int/medical_devices/innovation/MedDRAintroguide_version14_0_March2011.pdf

» Klepper MJ. MedDRA-An Introduction [Internet]. 2005 [cited 2012 May 24]. Available from: http://www.rti.org/pubs/meddra_intro.pdf

» Regulatory Harmonization - ICH : International Federation of Pharmaceutical Manufacturers & Associations [Internet]. [cited 2012 May 29]. Available from: http://www.ifpma.org/quality/regulatory-harmonization.html

Medicare Provider Analysis and Review (MedPAR)

» MedicareProviderAnalysisandReviewFile [Internet]. 2012 [cited 2013 Jan 30]. Available from: http://www.cms.gov/Research-Statistics-Data-and-Systems/Files-for-Order/IdentifiableDataFiles/MedicareProviderAnalysisandReviewFile.html

» Medpac Report to Congress: Chapter 3 Hospital inpatient and outpatient services [Internet]. 2012 Mar. Available from: http://www.medpac.gov/chapters/Mar12_Ch03.pdf

» MEDPAR Expanded Modified Record [Internet]. 2003 [cited 2013 Feb 2]. Available from: ftp://ftp.cdc.gov/pub/health_statistics/nchs/datalinkage/cms/medpar_snf.pdf

» ResDAC [Internet]. [cited 2013 Jan 29]. Available from: http://www.resdac.org/

Minimum Data Set (MDS)

» Giannangelo K. Healthcare Code Sets, Clinical Terminologies, and Classification Systems. 2nd ed. AHIMA; 2009.

» National Committee on Vital and Health Statistics [Internet]. [cited 2012 Sep 26]. Available from: http://www.cdc.gov/nchs/data/ncvhs/ncvhs89.pdf

National Database of Nursing Quality Indicators (NDNQI)

» ANA Indicator History [Internet]. [cited 2013 Aug 13]. Available from: http://www.nursingworld.org/MainMenuCategories/ThePracticeofProfessionalNursing/PatientSafetyQuality/Research-Measurement/The-National-Database/Nursing-Sensitive-Indicators_1/ANA-Indicator-History

» Montalvo I. The National Database of Nursing Quality Indicators® (NDNQI®). OJIN [Internet]. 2007 Sep [cited 2012 Aug 6];12(3). Available from: http://nursingworld.org/MainMenuCategories/ANAMarketplace/ANAPeriodicals/OJIN/TableofContents/Volume122007/No3Sept07/NursingQualityIndicators.aspx

» NDNQI Nursing Quality [Internet]. [cited 2012 Aug 9]. Available from: http://www.nursingquality.org/

» The Donabedian model of patient safety [Internet]. 2005 [cited 2012 Aug 9]. Available from: http://www.ahrq.gov/research/findings/final-reports/medteam/figure2.html

National Drug Codes (NDC)

» Hoyt RE, Yoshihashi A. Medical Informatics: Practical Guide for Healthcare and Information Technology Professionals Fourth Edition. 4th ed. lulu.com; 2010.

» Research C for DE and. Drug Approvals and Databases - National Drug Code Directory [Internet]. [cited 2012 Feb 12]. Available from: http://www.fda.gov/Drugs/InformationOnDrugs/ucm142438.htm

National Hospital Ambulatory Medical Care Survey (NHAMCS)

» Duke University | Economics: NHAMCS [Internet]. [cited 2013 Jan 13]. Available from: http://econ.duke.edu/tcrdc/census-data/health/nhamcs

» NAMCS/NHAMCS - Ambulatory Health Care Data Homepage [Internet]. [cited 2013 Jan 3]. Available from: http://www.cdc.gov/nchs/ahcd.htm

National Hospital Care Survey (NHCS)

» CDC: National Health Care Surveys [Internet]. [cited 2013 Feb 4]. Available from: http://www.cdc.gov/nchs/dhcs.htm

» National Hospital Discharge Survey [Internet]. National Center for Health Statistics; 2012 [cited 2013 Feb 1]. Available from: ftp://ftp.cdc.gov/pub/Health_statistics/ NCHs/Dataset_Documentation/NHDS/NHDS_2010_Documentation.pdf

» NHCS - About the National Hospital Care Survey [Internet]. [cited 2013 Jan 20]. Available from: http://www.cdc.gov/nchs/nhcs.htm

National Surgical Quality Improvement Program (NSQIP)

» American College of Surgeons || ACS NSQIP [Internet]. [cited 2013 Feb 4]. Available from: http://site.acsnsqip.org/about/

» American College of Surgeons: Continuous Quality Improvement: Program Overview [Internet]. [cited 2013 Feb 3]. Available from: http://www.facs.org/cqi/outcomes.html

» Fuchshuber PR, Greif W, Tidwell CR, Klemm MS, Frydel C, Wali A, et al. The power of the National Surgical Quality Improvement Program--achieving a zero pneumonia rate in general surgery patients. Perm J [Internet]. 2012 [cited 2013 Feb 2];16(1):39–45. Available from: http://www.ncbi.nlm.nih.gov/pubmed/22529758

National Trauma Data Bank (NTDB)

» American College of Surgeons Trauma Programs: National Trauma Data Bank [Internet]. [cited 2013 Jan 22]. Available from: http://www.facs.org/trauma/ntdb/

» American College of Surgeons: Trauma Programs: NTDB: National Sample Program [Internet]. [cited 2013 Jan 22]. Available from: http://www.facs.org/trauma/ntdb/nsp.html

» Champion HR, Copes WS, Sacco WJ, Lawnick MM, Keast SL, Bain LW Jr, et al. The Major Trauma Outcome Study: establishing national norms for trauma care. J Trauma [Internet]. 1990 Nov [cited 2012 Jan 13];30(11):1356–65. Available from: http://www.ncbi.nlm.nih.gov/pubmed/2231804

» National Trauma Data Bank - Home [Internet]. [cited 2013 Jan 24]. Available from: https://www.ntdbdatacenter.com/Default.aspx

National Vital Statistics System (NVSS)

» Attacks NC on T. The 9/11 Commission Report: Final Report of the National Commission on Terrorist Attacks Upon the United States. First Edition. W. W. Norton & Company; 2004.

» CDC - National Center for Health Statistics [Internet]. [cited 2013 Mar 23]. Available from: http://www.cdc.gov/nchs/index.htm

» Hetzel AM. U.S. Vital Statistics System, Major Activities and Developments, 1950-1995 [Internet]. Centers for Disease Control and Prevention/National Center for Health Statistics; 1997 [cited 2013 Mar 15]. Available from: http://www.cdc.gov/nchs/data/misc/usvss.pdf

» Michael J. Siri and Daniel L. Cork, Rapporteurs; Committee on National Statistics; National Research Council. Vital Statistics:Summary of a Workshop. Washington, D.C.: The National Academies Press; 2009.

Outcome and Assessment Information Set (OASIS)

» Giannangelo K. Healthcare Code Sets, Clinical Terminologies, and Classification Systems. 2nd ed. AHIMA; 2009.

» HAVEN [Internet]. 2013 [cited 2012 Oct 15]. Available from: http://www.cms.gov/Medicare/Quality-Initiatives-Patient-Assessment-Instruments/OASIS/HAVEN.html

» Home Health Quality Initiative OASIS User Manuals [Internet]. 2013 [cited 2012 Oct 16]. Available from: http://www.cms.gov/Medicare/Quality-Initiatives-Patient-Assessment-Instruments/HomeHealthQualityInits/HHQIOASISUserManual.html

PatientsLikeMe

» Cedarbaum JM, Stambler N, Malta E, Fuller C, Hilt D, Thurmond B, et al. The ALS-FRS-R: a revised ALS functional rating scale that incorporates assessments of respiratory function. BDNF ALS Study Group (Phase III). J. Neurol. Sci. 1999 Oct 31;169(1-2):13–21.

» Brownstein CA, Brownstein JS, Williams DS, Wicks P, Heywood JA. The power of social networking in medicine. Nat Biotech [Internet]. 2009 Oct [cited 2012 Jun 23];27(10):888–90. Available from: http://www.nature.com/nbt/journal/v27/n10/full/nbt1009-888.html

» Frost J, Okun S, Vaughan T, Heywood J, Wicks P. Patient-reported Outcomes as a Source of Evidence in Off-Label Prescribing: Analysis of Data From PatientsLikeMe. Journal of Medical Internet Research [Internet]. 2011 Jan 21 [cited 2012 Jun 22];13(1):e6. Available from: http://www.jmir.org/2011/1/e6/

» Frost JH, Massagli MP, Wicks P, Heywood J. How the Social Web Supports Patient Experimentation with a New Therapy: The demand for patient-controlled and patient-centered informatics. AMIA Annu Symp Proc [Internet]. 2008 [cited 2012 Jun 20];2008:217–21. Available from: http://www.ncbi.nlm.nih.gov/pmc/articles/PMC2656086/

» Live better, together! | PatientsLikeMe [Internet]. PatientsLikeMe. [cited 2012 Jun 20]. Available from: http://www.patientslikeme.com/

» Wicks P. The Patients Like Me Journey [Internet]. Eurodis; 2009 [cited 2012 Jun 21]. Available from: http://www.eurordis.org/IMG/pdf/amm_09/2-7_Eurordis%20PatientsLikeMe.pdf

» Wicks P, Massagli M, Frost J, Brownstein C, Okun S, Vaughan T, et al. Sharing Health Data for Better Outcomes on PatientsLikeMe. Journal of Medical Internet Research [Internet]. 2010 Jun 14 [cited 2012 Jun 22];12(2):e19. Available from: http://www.jmir.org/2010/2/e19/

» Wicks P, Massagli MP, Wolf C, Heywood J. Measuring function in advanced ALS: validation of ALSFRS-EX extension items. Eur. J. Neurol. [Internet]. 2009 Mar [cited 2012 Jun 21];16(3):353–9. Available from: http://www.ncbi.nlm.nih.gov/pubmed/19364363

» Wicks P, Vaughan TE, Massagli MP, Heywood J. Accelerated clinical discovery using self-reported patient data collected online and a patient-matching algorithm. Nat Biotech [Internet]. 2011 May [cited 2012 Jun 23];29(5):411–4. Available from: http://www.nature.com/nbt/journal/v29/n5/full/nbt.1837.html

Pediatric Quality Measures Program (PQMP)

» Child and Adolescent Health and Health Care Quality: Measuring What Matters [Internet]. [cited 2013 Feb 2]. Available from: http://www.nap.edu/openbook.php?record_id=13084

» Children's Health Insurance Program Reauthorization Act (CHIPRA) | Medicaid.gov [Internet]. [cited 2013 May 3]. Available from: http://medicaid.gov/Medicaid-CHIP-Program-Information/By-Topics/Childrens-Health-Insurance-Program-CHIP/CHIPRA.html

» CHIPRA Pediatric Quality Measures Program [Internet]. [cited 2013 May 2]. Available from: http://www.ahrq.gov/policymakers/chipra/pqmpback.html

» Quality Portal [Internet]. [cited 2013 Mar 13]. Available from: http://www.childhealthdata.org/browse/qualityportal

Prescription Drug Monitoring Programs (PDMPs)

» Alliance of States with Prescription Monitoring Programs | Promoting Public Health and Safety [Internet]. [cited 2012 Nov 20]. Available from: http://www.pmpalliance.org/

» Clark T, Eadie J, Kreiner P, Strickler G. Prescription Drug Monitoring Programs: An Assessment of the Evidence for Best Practices [Internet]. Center of Excellence Heller School for Social Policy and Management, Brandeis University; 2012. Available from: http://www.pewhealth.org/reports-analysis/reports/prescription-drug-moni-toring-programs-an-assessment-of-the-evidence-for-best-practices-85899418404

» Mostashari F, Clark W. Action Plan for Improving Access to Prescription Drug Mon-itoring Programs through Health Information Technology [Internet]. Department of Health and Human Services☐The Behavioral Health Coordinating Committee; 2011. Available from: http://www.healthit.gov/sites/default/files/rules-regula-tion/063012-final-action-plan-clearance.pdf

» Pew Charitable Trusts: Health Initiatives [Internet]. [cited 2012 Nov 23]. Available from: http://www.pewhealth.org/reports-analysis/reports/prescription-drug-moni-toring-programs-an-assessment-of-the-evidence-for-best-practices-85899418404

» Substance Abuse and Mental Health Services Administration [Internet]. [cited 2012 Nov 20]. Available from: http://www.samhsa.gov/

Resource-Based Relative Value Scale (RBRVS)

» Braun P, McCall N. Methodological Concerns with the Medicare RBRVS Payment System and Recommendations for Additional Study [Internet]. Available from: http://www.medpac.gov/documents/Aug11_Methodology_RBRVS_contractor.pdf

» History of the RBRVS [Internet]. American Medical Association. [cited 2012 Apr 1]. Available from: https://www.ama-assn.org/ama/pub/physician-resources/solu-tions-managing-your-practice/coding-billing-insurance/medicare/the-resource-based-relative-value-scale/history-of-rbrvs.page

» AC47:12-P-060:1C47:12-P-060:10/12

RxNorm

» Bennett CC. Utilizing RxNorm to support practical computing applications: Captur-ing medication history in live electronic health records. Journal of Biomedical Infor-matics [Internet]. 2012 Aug [cited 2012 Oct 26];45(4):634–41. Available from: http://www.sciencedirect.com/science/article/pii/S153204641200041X

» Giannangelo K. Healthcare Code Sets, Clinical Terminologies, and Classification Systems. 2nd ed. AHIMA; 2009.

» Hoyt RE, Yoshihashi A. Medical Informatics: Practical Guide for Healthcare and Information Technology Professionals Fourth Edition. 4th ed. lulu.com; 2010.

» RxNorm [Internet]. [cited 2012 Oct 27]. Available from: http://www.nlm.nih.gov/research/umls/rxnorm/

» Ryan S, McKinney F. NIST NCPDP Analysis – RxNorm Support Assessment [Internet]. 1st American Systems and Services LLC; 2011 [cited 2012 Oct 26]. Available from: http://healthcare.nist.gov/resources/docs/FirstAmerican/NIST_NCPDPRxNormSupportAssessment.pdf

Society for Thoracic Surgeons General Thoracic Surgery Database (STS GTSD)

» Jacobs JP, Edwards FH, Shahian DM, Haan CK, Puskas JD, Morales DLS, et al. Successful linking of the Society of Thoracic Surgeons adult cardiac surgery database to Centers for Medicare and Medicaid Services Medicare data. Ann. Thorac. Surg. 2010 Oct;90(4):1150–1156; discussion 1156–1157.

» STS National Database | STS [Internet]. [cited 2012 Jul 7]. Available from: http://www.sts.org/national-database

» Wimer P. Evolution of the Society of Thoracic Surgeons National Cardiac Surgery Database. The Journal of Lancaster General Hospital [Internet]. 2009 Fall [cited 2012 Jul 5];4(3). Available from: http://www.jlgh.org/JLGH/media/Journal-LGH-Media-Library/Past%20Issues/Volume%204%20-%20Issue%203/Wimerfall09.pdf

Standardized Nursing Languages (SNLs)

» Hebda TL, Czar P. Handbook of Informatics for Nurses and Healthcare Professionals. 4th ed. Prentice Hall; 2008.

» International N. Nursing Diagnoses: Definitions and Classification 2012-14. 9th ed. Wiley-Blackwell; 2011.

» Lee E, Park H, Nam M, Whyte J. Identification and Comparison of Interventions Performed by Korean School Nurses and U.S. School Nurses Using the Nursing Interventions Classification (NIC). The Journal of School Nursing [Internet]. 2010 Dec

2 [cited 2012 Dec 13];27(2):93–101. Available from: http://www.nasn.org/PolicyAd-vocacy/PositionPapersandReports/NASNPositionStatementsFullView/tabid/462/ArticleId/48/Standardized-Nursing-Languages-Revised-June-2012

» Ozbolt JG, Saba VK. A brief history of nursing informatics in the United States of America. Nurs Outlook [Internet]. 2008 Oct [cited 2012 Dec 11];56(5):199–205.e2. Available from: http://www.ncbi.nlm.nih.gov/pubmed/18922268

Systematized Nomenclature of Medicine-Clinical Terms (SNOMED CT)

» Giannangelo K. Healthcare Code Sets, Clinical Terminologies, and Classification Systems. 2nd ed. AHIMA; 2009.

» Hoyt RE, Yoshihashi A. Medical Informatics: Practical Guide for Healthcare and Information Technology Professionals Fourth Edition. 4th ed. lulu.com; 2010.

» Lehmann, H. P., Abbott, P. A., Roderer, N. K., Rothschild, A., Mandell, S., Ferrer, J. A., Miller, R. E., & Ball, M. J. (2006). Aspects of electronic health record systems. (2nd ed.). New York, NY: Springer.

» SNOMED CT: The Language of Electronic Health Records [Internet]. NHS-UK; 2010 [cited 2012 Feb 15]. Available from: http://www.connectingforhealth.nhs.uk/system-sandservices/data/uktc/training/snobrochure.pdf

TNM (Tumor, Node, Metastasis) Classification

» Cancer Staging Fact Sheet - National Cancer Institute [Internet]. [cited 2012 May 17]. Available from: http://www.cancer.gov/cancertopics/factsheet/detection/staging

» TNM History, Evolution and Milestones [Internet]. [cited 2012 Apr 16]. Available from: http://webcache.googleusercontent.com/search?q=cache:foa7V-deZGlEJ:www.uicc.org/system/files/private/History_Evolution_Milestones_0.pdf+&cd=1&hl=en&ct=clnk&gl=us&client=firefox-a

» Union for International Cancer Control [Internet]. [cited 2012 May 10]. Available from: http://www.uicc.org/about-uicc

Unified Medical Language System (UMLS)

» UMLS [Internet]. [cited 2012 Nov 2]. Available from: http://www.nlm.nih.gov/research/umls/about_umls.html

» UMLS® Reference Manual [Internet]. 2009 [cited 2012 Nov 2]. Available from: http://www.ncbi.nlm.nih.gov/books/NBK9676/

Uniform Ambulatory Care Data Set (UACDS)

» Kanaan SB. NCVHS 1949-1999 - A History [Internet]. [cited 2012 Oct 1]. Available from: http://www.ncvhs.hhs.gov/50history.htm

» National Committee on Vital and Health Statistics [Internet]. [cited 2012 Sep 26]. Available from: http://www.cdc.gov/nchs/data/ncvhs/nchvs89.pdf

» Unequal Treatment: Confronting Racial and Ethnic Disparities in Health Care - Institute of Medicine [Internet]. 2002 [cited 2012 Sep 25]. Available from: http://www.iom.edu/Reports/2002/Unequal-Treatment-Confronting-Racial-and-Ethnic-Disparities-in-Health-Care.aspx

Uniform Hospital Discharge Data Set (UHDDS)

» Giannangelo K. Healthcare Code Sets, Clinical Terminologies, and Classification Systems. 2nd ed. AHIMA; 2009.

» Kanaan SB. NCVHS 1949-1999 - A History [Internet]. [cited 2012 Oct 1]. Available from: http://www.ncvhs.hhs.gov/50history.htm

» NCVHS Report on Core Health Data Elements [Internet]. [cited 2012 Oct 2]. Available from: http://www.ncvhs.hhs.gov/ncvhsr1.htm

United Network for Organ Sharing (UNOS)

» Interrelationships.pdf [Internet]. [cited 2013 Jan 11]. Available from: https://cignalifesource.com/media/Interrelationships.pdf

» OPTN: Organ Procurement and Transplantation Network [Internet]. U. S. Department of Health & Human Services. [cited 2013 Jan 11]. Available from: http://optn.transplant.hrsa.gov/data/about/OPTNDatabase.asp

» Public Law 98-507: National Organ Transplant Act. 42 USC [Internet]. 1984 [cited 2013 Jan 13]. Available from: http://history.nih.gov/research/downloads/PL98-507.pdf

» UNOS | Donation & Transplantation | History [Internet]. [cited 2013 Jan 10]. Available from: http://www.unos.org/donation/index.php?topic=history

United States Health Information Knowledgebase (USHIK) and Meaningful Use (MU)

» Fitzmaurice JM. USHIK: A Meaningful Use One-Stop Shop [Internet]. 2012 [cited 2013 Feb 21]. Available from: http://www.healthit.gov/sites/default/files/hitsc_111212fitzm.pdf

» Fitzmaurice M, Barnes R, Donnelly J. AHRQ 2011 Annual Conference, Slide Presentation [Internet]. 2011 [cited 2013 Feb 24]. Available from: http://www.ahrq.gov/legacy/about/annualconf11/fitzmaurice_barnes_donnelly/fitzmauricebarnesdonnelly.htm

» Halamka J. Life as a Healthcare CIO: A First Look at Meaningful Use Stage 2 [Internet]. Life as a Healthcare CIO. 2012 [cited 2013 Feb 24]. Available from: http://geekdoctor.blogspot.com/2012/02/first-look-at-meaningful-use-stage-2.html

» Meaningful Use (FAQs) [Internet]. Agency for Healthcare Research and Quality. [cited 2013 Feb 25]. Available from: http://ushik.ahrq.gov/help/MeaningfulUse/faq?system=mu

» Meaningful_Use [Internet]. CMS.gov. 2013 [cited 2013 Feb 24]. Available from: https://www.cms.gov/Regulations-and-Guidance/Legislation/EHRIncentivePrograms/Meaningful_Use.html

Universal Medical Device Nomenclature System (UMDNS)

» ECRI Institute [Internet]. [cited 2012 Dec 7]. Available from: https://www.ecri.org/Pages/default.aspx

» ECRI Institute Adds 4,000 New Terms to Universal Medical Device Nomenclature SystemTM [Internet]. [cited 2012 Dec 6]. Available from: http://www.prnewswire.com/news-releases/ecri-institute-adds-4000-new-terms-to-universal-medical-device-nomenclature-system-98022584.html

» Halamka J. Life as a Healthcare CIO: Standards for Naming Medical Devices [Internet]. Life as a Healthcare CIO. 2010 [cited 2012 Dec 7]. Available from: http://geekdoctor.blogspot.com/2010/07/standards-for-naming-medical-devices.html

» 2012AA UMD Source Information [Internet]. U.S. National Library of Medicine. [cited 2012 Dec 6]. Available from: http://www.nlm.nih.gov/research/umls/sourcereleasedocs/current/UMD/index.html

About the Authors

Katherine S. Rowell, MS, MHA

Kathy Rowell is co-founder and principal of Katherine S. Rowell & Associates and HealthDataViz, a Boston firm that specializes in helping healthcare organizations organize, design, and present visual displays of data to inform their decisions and stimulate effective action. She advises providers, payers, policymakers and regulatory agencies how to align systems, design reports, and develop staff to communicate healthcare data clearly.

She made crucial contributions to the establishment of the Massachusetts General Hospital Codman Center for Clinical Effectiveness and the launching of the National Surgical Quality Improvement Program (300+ participating hospitals throughout the U.S. and Canada). A much-in-demand speaker at Grand Rounds and healthcare conferences, Rowell has published numerous high-profile articles, and Unleash Your Inner Healthcare Data, her twice-monthly newsletter, has passionate subscribers all over the world. Her clients, drawn from leading national and international healthcare organizations, include the Cleveland Clinic, Partners Healthcare, Baylor Healthcare, the World Health Organization, and the Children's Hospital Association. They and hundreds of other companies, organizations, and individuals seek out her public and private workshops, in-house training sessions, and private consulting services to learn the best practices of data visualization for healthcare professionals and other stakeholders.

Kathy holds a BS in Business Management and a Master's in Health Administration from the University of New Hampshire, and an MS from Dartmouth Medical School. A former member of the faculty of Brandeis University's Medical Informatics Graduate Program, Kathy continues to serve on its Advisory Committee. She is a recipient of the prestigious Partners in Excellence Award for leadership and innovation.

Kathy lives in Brookline, Massachusetts, with husband Bret, daughter Anne, adorable pup Juno, and way cool boat "Visualize."

Ann Cutrell, M.S., R.Ph.

Ann Cutrell is an expert in the design and implementation of integrated management software that tracks, organizes, presents, and applies data to support optimum clinical outcomes and control costs, while helping providers comply with government healthcare initiatives.

Cutrell's success at both the theoretical and the practical sides of software creation and use have built on her extensive experience managing a private company specializing in pharmaceuticals and services for respiratory-ailment patients, where she worked with physicians and pharmacy benefit managers, and supervised staff in both institutional and home settings to enhance disease- and care-management. Her broad and deep knowledge of the field combined with her front-line contribution to efficient, proactive healthcare delivery have enabled her to effectively support clients as they gather, display, and interpret industry statistics and results in ways that will lead to the most practical and effective healthcare decisions possible.

Ann Cutrell holds a BS in Pharmacy from Duquesne University, and an MS in Health and Medical Informatics at Brandeis University, where she was a student of Katherine Rowell. She is a licensed pharmacist (Pennsylvania), a triathlete and marathoner, and a tireless advocate for the developmentally disabled.

CPSIA information can be obtained
at www.ICGtesting.com
Printed in the USA
LVHW071628150522
718836LV00002B/22